ROSINA FASCHING – TEA FUNGUS KOMBUCHA

ROSINA FASCHING

Tea Fungus Kombucha

The Natural Remedy
and its Significance in Cases of Cancer and other Metabolic Diseases

With nine photographs in color and a topography of the iris

PUBLISHING HOUSE ENNSTHALER, STEYR

9th extended and revised edition 1995

ISBN 3 85068 231 5

TABLE OF CONTENTS

PREFACE

The on hand entitled publication "TEA FUNGUS KOMBUCHA" is based on decades of observation along with my practical experience as a physician and cancer researcher. I would also like this publication to be viewed as a contribution to the entire complex concerning the cancer problem. My methods for early diagnosis of cancer and precancerous conditions by means of the iris diagnostics and blood dyeing as well as the methods of treatment that I have acquired through work and experience shall be made available to those who still associate cancer with intolerable suffering, pain und inevitable death.

Even though as a physician I make use of "outsiders' methods", it is because I am convinced that only a combination *of all forces* and *all knowledge* can lead us to our goal in the problem of cancer. And the goal can only be to diagnose this disease in the early stages of its development and treat it accordingly. Therefore, in order to fight cancer successfully, the first thing we need is a sensible attitude whose line of reasoning is not clouded by emotions. Means for an early diagnosis of cancer – such as the diagnosis of the iris – are rejected by a majority of physicians who are not prepared to accept the findings based on this auxiliary method. If cancer is indeed a malignant malfunction which has eluded the organism, the question arises: what are the reasons for such a derailment, and where does the first wrong impulse originate from?

In this situation the practitioner is faced with only one question: how should he diagnose, how should he cure?

Moreover it is time for theoreticians and practitioners to understand that cancer is nothing special, but that tumors are to be considered as only one among many chronic metabolic diseases. The initial phase of the tumor is triggered by a disturbed metabolism; therefore this is where treatment and prophylaxis must begin. As long as academic medicine is incapable of preventing cancer by means of inoculation, "healing cancer" will remain utopian; but we do have possibilities to help even at an advanced stage of cancer. Helping means prolonging life under bearable conditions, and eliminating complications, anxiety and fear.

In using the tea fungus Kombucha, colicines and other biological remedies I see my therapy in cases of cancer and other chronic diseases as an alternative method, which is valid until it is possible to immunize the healthy person against cancer through inoculation.

The viruses recently discovered by Drs. R. C. Gallo (USA) and 8L. Montagnier (Paris), and previously by several other cancer researchers (e.g. v. Brehmer, Scheller, Enderlein and myself) are identical. In this case one and the same thing has only been interpreted in different ways. There have been world-wide endeavors toward an immunization, i.e. toward finding an effective vaccine, and I am confident that it will be discovered. Considering the fact, however, that between the discovery of the hepatitis-B-virus and the development of an efficient vaccine no less than 16 years elapsed, we should be grateful to make use of an alternative therapy.

This booklet is meant to familiarize the reader with the results of my scientific research as well as my practical experience and also to reintroduce a natural remedy which has fallen into oblivion, but which was popular and highly esteemed for centuries.

Rudolf Sklenar, M. D.
Lich/Upper Hessia, November, 1984.

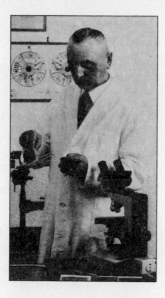

Letter from Dr. Sklenar
dated 18 April 1986:

Dr. med. Rudolf Sklenar

Garbenteicher Straße 23
6302 Lich, 18 April 1986

During the more than 30 years I have been working as a general practitioner, I have been using for therapy the beverage prepared from the tea fungus Kombucha, and also the drops of the Kombucha concentrate, preferably combining it with coli preparations to cure intestinal disturbances.

The therapeutics based on Kombucha produced good therapeutical results in cases of metabolic diseases, also with those of a chronic nature. Good results were achieved also with cancer diseases in various stages. In no instance undesired side or late effects caused by a treatment with these therapeutics were ascertainable.

Dr. med. Rudolf Sklenar

INTRODUCTION

The 2nd edition of this book has been enlarged by essential information, which is important for the consumer. Since the publication of the first edition in 1985 I have received countless reports on therapeutic experience and success letters of thanks and inquiries. Therefore it seems necessary to answer, in this place, questions of general interest.

Being the collaborator and niece of Dr. med. Rudolf Sklenar, I have been able to acquire his method of diagnosis and therapy as well as his nearly 40 years of practical experience with the tea fungus Kombucha. I became a wittness of astounding therapeutic success and have always been astonished by his "simple" methods at low expense with which he discovered even hidden diseases and cured them successfully.

All my knowledge, which I make available to the general public by means of this book, I owe to him.

I note with pleasure the growing interest within the medical profession in applying the scientific findings of Dr. Sklenar and prescribing Kombucha products to thankful patients.

Well, on one hand the tea fungus enjoys growing popularity, but on the other hand recently lack of assurance and information have been perceived. Furthermore, tea fungus and tea fungus imitations from undeclared sources are brought on the market without control. Analyses disclosed a. o. substances that were not from the tea fungus and sometimes of a rather strange nature.

The boom of the Kombucha produces some strange phenomena in Southern Germany and in Austria: the tea fungus is named after its origin tea of algae or "Riementangtee" and is sold by the name of "Kombucha" or "Fungus of China". Its originality is suspect. From this point of view it has become necessary to advise against preparing the beverage by oneself and to refrain from tea fungus cultures and products respectively from dubious origin. Furthermore, some rather strange "directions for use" are circulated which are of no service to anyone in this matter.

One of Dr. Sklenar's experiences is especially important for diabetics: the beverage of Kombucha is not suitable for them; but they can use some other extract; its extraction and production are subject to the original recipe and method according to Dr. Sklenar.

Please note that reducing the amount of sugar for the preparation of the starting material is no solution, because the process of fermentation and transformation of the components would result, as ascertained, in the reduction of the wholesome and natural components of the beverage of Kombucha. Surrogates of sugar are entirely inapt; honey – as well as some brands of herb tea – proved to be a failure, because they contain ethereal oils. In any case on a long-term basis this would result in a transformation of the fungus culture.

So it is recommended to remember Samuel Hahnemann, the founder of the classical homeopathy, who told his pupils: "Copy it, but copy it exactly!"

Therefore it is of great importance for all tea fungus consumers that they follow exactly the directions for growing the fungus cultivations, preparing and applying the beverage according to the decades of experience of the physician Dr. Sklenar.

For all those reasons I can recommend only the original products "Kombucha nach Dr. Sklenar" (Kombucha according to Dr. Sklenar), because the producer the firm of "Dr. med. Sklenar Bio-Produkte GmbH" in Dorsten/Bochum fabricates according to original recipes, avails of Dr. Sklenar's experience and its fabrication of the Kombucha products is regularly controlled by certificated food chemists.

The firm of "Dr. med. Sklenar Bio-Produkte GmbH" in Dorsten/Bochum have obtained the licence for products of Kombucha according to Dr. Sklenar, which can be sold as food of a special kind.

I would like to remind you of Hippocrates' advice:

"Your remedies shall be your food and your food shall be your remedies."[1]

---

1 In: Prof. Dr. G. Enderlein 1955, p. 81.

Part I

The Tea Fungus Kombucha . . .

History, Discovery and Geographical Spread

For centuries the tea fungus Kombucha has enjoyed great popularity as a natural remedy. Already in ancient China, during the reign of the Tsin Dynasty in 221 B.C., fungi were seen as a means for attaining immortality. They were the source of magic power. The most famous one is the "Divine Che". *Ganoderma japonicus Lloyd,* which is the same as "Divine Che" (Ling-tche), is still used in southern China for the treatment of chronic gastritis.[1] Medical history also contains reports about a Korean doctor named *Kombu,* who was called to Japan to treat the Emperor Inkyo. The year 414 is probably the date when the "Che of Kombu" reached Japan. Quite obviously there was no discovery of the fungus in the traditional sense, since it is neither the final product of a pharmaceutical process, nor the discovery of a researcher in his laboratory, but a successful natural symbiosis of primitive organisms.

From Korea, Japan, China and India the fungus spread via Russia into the countries of Eastern Europe, where it enjoys great popularity on account of its salutary effect in the treatment of metabolic diseases. Up to World War II Kombucha was to be found in almost every household. When the war brought about a shortage of black tea and sugar, which are essential for the preservation of the fungus, it lost its popularity and fell into oblivion. Only occasional hints in outdated literature point out the existence of this formerly popular natural remedy. Among others, *Hans Irion* in his "Lehrgang für Drogistenfachschule"[2] (Instructions for Druggists' School) reports about the tea fungus Fungus japonicus,

---

1 Cf. "Illustrated History of Medicine in Nine Volumes", Volume 1. Published by Andreas & Andreas, Salzburg, 1980, p. 81

2 Irion, Hans (Ed.): Lehrgang für Drogistenfachschule in 4 Bänden. Volume 2: Botany – Lore of Drugs. Published by Rudolf Müller, Eberswalde-Berlin-Leipzig 1942, p. 405

Fungojapon Kombucha, Indo-Japanese tea fungus. Literature also knows it by the names "Pichia fermentans", "Cembuya orientalis", "Combuchu", "Tschambucco", "Volga spring", "Mo-Gû", "Champignon de longue vie", "tea kvas", "Kwassan", "Hongo", "Haipao", "Kocha Kinoko", "Red Tea Fungus" etc.

In the 1950s Kombucha came to be the favorite drink of Italian 'high snobiety'. When somebody, for some base reason or other, declared that it was cancer-inducing, it lost its allure. Research in Switzerland, however, proved the exact opposite in 1960: The tea fungus is as wholesome as, say, yoghurt, and it is available in every pharmacy in Franconian Switzerland under the registered name tea fungus Mo-Gû. The pharmacist M. Bergold reports: "The delicious beverage resembling fruit wine made of the tea fungus Mo-Gû exercises a soothing effect in cases of constipation and detoxicates to a great extent pathogenic intestinal bacteria."

According to extensive investigations by famous biologists the beverage prepared from the tea fungus is a natural product deriving from the fermentation process with a high vitamin content that influences very positively the metabolic process of the human body and serves predominantly the prevention of intestinal diseases and their consecutive symptoms.[1]

In 1964 *Rudolf Sklenar, M. D.*, first published his practical experience with the tea fungus Kombucha gained in the course of many years.[2] Since that time Kombucha[3] has enjoyed a renascence and is on the way toward regaining its previous popularity.

1 Bergold, M. (pharmacist): Teepilz Mo-Gu (Informationsblatt der Waischenfelder Apotheke), Waischenfeld, Franconian Switzerland.

2 Dr. med. Sklenar, Rudolf in: Sonderdruck aus Erfahrungsheilkunde. Zeitschrift für die tägliche Praxis. Volume XIII, issue 3. Karl F. Haug Verlag. Ulm,/Donau, 1964.

3 KOMBUCHA® according to Dr. Sklenar (Kombucha® nach Dr. Sklenar) is an internationally protected trade mark.

The Fungus

The uncontaminated fungus cultures constitute a natural symbiosis of Saccharomyces ludwigii, Saccharomyces apiculatus varieties, Bacterium xylinum, Bacterium xylinoides, Bacterium gluconicum, Schizosaccharomyces pombe, Acetobacter ketogenum, Torula varieties, Pichia fermentans and other enzymes.

In contrast to genuine ferments, these mixed cultures do not produce any spores, but multiply exclusively in a vegetative manner by sprouting. Today the Kombucha beverage is already produced industrially, which guarantees protection against infections as well as high quality.

Components and Effect

The symbiotic partners of the Kombucha fungus thrive in the nutritive broth. Through their organic processes they ferment the sugar, resulting in the production of various metabolic substances, which constitute part of the beverage. Among these mainly glucuronic acid, lactic acid and various vitamins that are considered beneficial. The average alcohol content is a mere 0.5 %; Zeller notes that the alcohol content is not even $1/4$ percent, since the bacteria manage the transformation into gluconic acid.[1]

The carbonic acid gives the drink its refreshing effect, so that people describe it as a veritable thirst quencher. Not to be forgotten, its aromatic components produced by Kombucha's symbiosis constitute the aroma so typical of the Kombucha beverage.

Furthermore Zeller reports: "The culture consists of a thick, gelatinous skin which can produce best in tea, because latter contains the purines necessary for the growth of the fungus. It has not yet been proved scientifically, whether or not the fungus absorbes the coffeine, but what strikes one is that organisms sensitive to tea do not show any negative reactions when absorbing the kwas of the tea added."[2]

At the same time Zeller warns against using various sorts or mixtures of tea, because neither the good taste, nor the functional capacity or viability ... can be achieved with infusions.[3]

1 A. P. Zeller: Das Reich der Hausfrau. Ensslin-Druck, Reutlingen, 1924.
2 Ibidem.
3 Ibidem.

It turned out that when using various sorts of tea and honey respectively or other surrogates of sugar, the fungus cultures are modified by the ethereal oils and the "balance" of the symbionts of fungus (yeasts and bacteria) become displaced. In 1942 Hans Orion warned "against using so-called offshoots … because they stem either from the well-known mother of vinegar or from worn-out fungi, contaminated by germs from the air."[1]

The pharmacist Bergold recommended: "Older fungi are contaminated by mould fungi of various kinds, thus no longer in a perfect condition and therefore need to be removed."[2]

Do check the composition of the fungus culture (source of supply) and its purity, since recently tea fungus imitations (fakes) of doubtful origin have been thrown on the market.

To be sure it would be a misconception to believe that a few isolated components of the Kombucha fungus might have the same beneficial influence on the human organism, because the real beverage is an inimitable composite, and only as such it exerts its manifold curative influence on man. Aristotle, the great philosopher of ancient Greece, already knew:

The whole is more than the sum of its parts.

Despite a number of analyses the secret of this "divine Che" was not completely unraveled. There always remained a "sugar derivative of unknown composition from the category of gluconic acids". But all are agreed on the fact that the glucuronic acid contained therein effects a substantial detoxication of the organism. This is of such eminent importance for the human body because as a so-called 'coupled glucuronic acid' it forms compounds with metabolic waste products as well as substances alien to the body (drugs and poisons), and thus aids in detoxicating the organism. Moreover, glucuronic acid in compound form is a component of such vital polysaccharides as hyaluronic acid (basic component of the connective tissue), chondroitin sulfate (basic component of cartilage), mucoitinsulfuric acid (component of gastric mucous membranes and the vitreous body of the eye) and heparin.

---

1 Hans Orion 1942, p. 405.
2 M. Bergold, (pharmacist): Teepilz Mo-Gu (Informationsblatt der Waischenfelder Apotheke), Waischenfeld, Franconian Switzerland.

Besides, Kombucha contains lactic acid, and therefore displays an impeding effect toward a number of bacteria, mainly putrefactive bacteria of the intestine, which in the process are suppressed. Thus Kombucha also has antibiotic properties.

The beverage has a striking effect of invigorating the whole system of glands and enhancing metabolism. In cases of digestive troubles one or two glasses of Kombucha drunk on an empty stomach in the morning, after meals at noon and in the evening are a great help. The beverage introduces micro-organisms into the body which transform harmful substances such as uric acid and cholesterol into more soluble compounds, and thus remove them. In the sixties the "Waischenfelder Apotheke" recommended the tea fungus as follows "The ‚Tea Fungus Mo-Gû' is recommended, in the form of a daily beverage, as an excellent preventative and therapeutic remedy against metabolic diseases (gout, rheumatism, furunculosis), early arteriosclerosis and its accompaniments, against physical and mental fatigue (in cases of continuous overwork in agriculture, in sports), to stimulate the bowel function (constipation, obesity, sensation of repletion) and to increase the general state of health (insufficient sexual drive) and during convalescent periods."[1]

Moreover, Hans Orion recommended the use of the tea fungus in cases of furunculosis, high blood pressure, nervousness and symptoms of old age. He writes: "It is highly recommended also to sporting people and to mental workers. By activating the metabolism in the body excessive corpulence can be avoided or removed."[2]

Because of the purifying effect of this beverage and because of its capability to destroy harmful microorganisms Kombucha is a helpful biological "universal remedy" against various metabolic diseases, which does not produce unwanted side effects.

Kombucha's pH-(i.e. acidity) level of 3.0 is of utmost importance.

There seems to be great confusion concerning the preference of acid (lactic acid) und basic (alkaline) food respectively, and the pH value (value of hydrogenion concentration) has also caused irritation. The pH value is simply the value that indicates the degree of acidity of a liquid. The neutral point is 7; values below this point (6.9, 6.8 etc.) indicate an acid

1 M. Bergold, (pharmacist): Teepilz Mo-Gu (Informationsblatt der Waischenfelder Apotheke), Waischenfeld, Franconian Switzerland.

2 Hans Orion 1942, p. 405.

reaction; higher figures (7.1, 7.2 etc.) show basic (alkaline) reaction. In cases of alkaline reactions, for example the free negatively charged hydroxide ions are available in excess compared to the positively charged hydrogen ions.

The pH-level of blood both in a healthy and in a sick person is subject to wide fluctuations. For decades it was assumed to be constant (some people possibly still think so). In young years the pH-level of human blood is on the acid side, but over the years it becomes increasingly alkaline (basic). The limit for humans is 8.0, subject to variations toward acidity, about 6.0. Generally the pH-level should not rise above 7.5, as a level of 7.56 sets the stage for the development of tumors.

Based on their extensive research, Höpke and Schepelmann report in their book: "Beeinflussung des Tumorwachstums durch saure und basische Ernährung" (Influencing the growth of tumors by acidic and alkaline nutrition) "... acidic nutrition can have a retarding effect upon the development of tumors". In many circles one hears talk about hyperacidity ('acid rain' etc.). We can recommend Dr. Emil Scheller's book: "Krebsschutz durch Früherkennung und Ursachenbehandlung" (Prevention of Cancer by Early Diagnosis and Treatment of its Root Causes)[1], in which he explains the two isomeric variants of like components of lactic acid:

1. the optically active levogyral lactic acid (l-lactic acid)
2. the optically active dextrogyral lactic acid (d-lactic acid = tissue lactic acid in active, fatigued muscles) and
3. a mixture of the two:
   the optically inactive, racemic lactic acid (d-l-lactic acid = lactic fermentation within the cancerous growth).

Thus the lack of d-lactic acid in nutrition causes a disturbance of cellular respiration, the decomposition of sugar by fermentation, and the formation of d-l-lactic acid in the body tissue.

Lactic acid in the nutrition is entirely different to lactic acid in the tissue. There exists a contradiction in the fact that lactic acid in the tissue, which is a toxic substance, can be neutralized or decomposed by lactic acid in the nutrition.

Normally lactic acid is burned in the stomach to carbonic acid and water. In case the vesticular breathing is damaged or even destroyed, the lactic acid of the tissue can no longer be decomposed and thus is

1   Published by Humata, Harold S. Blume

18

deposited pathologically in the body. In such a case Kuhl affirms that it is possible to reduce the toxic lactic acid by giving to the body small or very small quantities of lactic acid.

Thus the disturbed balance of acid-base in the body can be reestablished according to points of view of isopathy: The same thing is replaced by the same thing – but in a different quantity.[1]

A complete vegetarian diet does not offer adequate protection because it tends to be alkaline; nutrition without lactic acid leads to chronic deficiency, because it alters the pH-level of the blood toward the alkaline side. Nutrition rich in lactic acid, however, besides manual labor, muscle exercise, sauna etc., promotes the excretion of wastes and produces lactic acid, which regulates the pH-level of the blood.

First samples of blood from the veins have shown Kombucha to have the effect of making the blood more acid.

It has been reported that with elderly people Kombucha has a rejuvenating effect, causing grey hair to grow in dark again, tightening the skin and enhancing the feeling of vitality and health. Moreover the regular sipping of Kombucha can keep the teeth healthy. As we know, the pH-level of saliva is determined by the pH-level of the blood and plays its part in the development of caries.

This should be reason enough to provide children with the Kombucha drink instead of the current sugary refreshment beverages.

Directions for Preparation of Kombucha at Home

Tea is to be prepared as usual – normally two litres. The basic recipe should be the following: for one litre of water take one teaspoonful of black tea and 100 to 125 g of sugar.

> Some people who can take black tea very well sometimes react to Kombucha with palpitations of the heart and nervousness. Under those circumstances one can substitute black tea by infusions for the liver, the nerves, for the stomach and the intestines and various other herb mixtures can be taken. But one needs to make sure that only herb mixtures are used that do not contain too high a level of ethereal oils. When preparing other types of infusions take two teaspoonsfuls of tea for one litre of water.

---

1 See Scheller

After this sugared infusion has cooled down to body temperature (about 36 degrees C), the liquid is poured into a glass container for 3 litres, the liquid of the fungus is added. Then place the fungus on top. Close the glass container with a layer of gauze to protect it against dust and insects, and fix it with a rubber band. Then place the glass on the cupboard.

After preparation the fungus can sink to the bottom. Do not move the glass. If the fungus stays on the bottom, a new fungus grows on the surface.

To develop and grow, the Kombucha needs rest, fresh air and, first of all, a lot of warmth (ca. 23 degrees C). This would be the ideal temperature. A scope of plus/minus five degrees has no influence, but a temperature of less than 14 or more then 30 degrees C should be avoided. In the first circumstance the fermentation is slowed down drastically and only the yeasts are well activated but not the bacteria of the fungus. If the temperature is too high, i. e. 29 degrees C and more, the activity of the bacteria increases and the fungus becomes mucoid.

One should not smoke in this room, because this encourages the growth of molds, but they can be removed with vinegar. After approximately eight to ten days, this depends on the acidity of the beverage, remove the fungus, filter off the liquid, fill it into bottles and put it into the refrigerator.

One should drink one or two glasses of Kombucha every day in the morning on an empty stomach, before lunch and before dinner. It tastes delicious, slightly sour, sparkling – nearly like a light Moselle.

One should start immediately to cultivate a new beverage as recommended above. Put about three fingers of the old liquid of the fungus (the prepared beverage of Kombucha) into the cleaned glass (acidification). Always remove old settlings. After several cultivations the fungus has become thicker. Since the top layer of the fungus is always the latest one, remove from time to time the bottom layer of the fungus.

It is well known that *Paracelsus* fermented all medical herbs this way and thus achieved his great therapeutic successes. In fact, this fermentation causes a breakdown of all substances and thus a multiplication (potentiation) of the effect.

If treated adequately, i.e. in the above-mentioned way, the fungus Kombucha gives you pleasure all your life. It was already *Samuel Hahnemann*, the father of the classical homeopathy, who recommended to his pupils:

Copy it, but copy it correctly!

Part II

... and Its Significance in the Treatment of Cancer

First of all we would like to point out the research results of the German physician *Dr. Valentin Köhler.* By means of glucuronic acid, which is one of Kombucha's components, he obtained surprising results in the treatment of clinically hopeless cases of cancer. He was able to note:

- no new metastases
- weight loss arrested, in some cases even reversed
- improvement of the general well-being
- no confinement to bed
- increased interest in the environment
- curtailment of analgetics (painkillers)
- decrease of coughing fits[1]

At the University of Munich Dr. Köhler's method of watering ailing trees with an admixture of glucuronic acid is being tested after he has pioneered it sucessfully.

The research of the German physician *Dr. Sklenar* is not restricted to an extract of the Kombucha fungus and goes even further. He draws experience from more than 30 years of practical application. To begin with, he noted the beneficial effect of the Kombucha beverage on patients suffering from metabolic disturbances. Today he is able to look back on a long series of successful treatment of serious afflictions such as precancerous ailments and cancer, with the help of the tea fungus. It was especially in the field of cancer therapy and prevention that Kombucha, in combination with colicines, has proved to be an extremely successful remedy, both on account of its cleansing and antibiotic properties.[2]

1 Valentin Köhler, M. D.: Glukuronsäure macht Krebspatienten Mut (Glucuronic Acid Gives New Hope to Cancer Patients) in the magazine "Ärztliche Praxis"/Issue 24, 1981, p. 887

2 Rudolf Sklenar, M. D.: Krebsdiagnose aus dem Blut und die Behandlung von Krebs und Präkanzerosen mit der Kombucha und Colipräparaten (Cancer Diagnosis through the Blood and the Treatment of Cancer and Pre-Cancerous Ailments by Means of Kombucha and Colicines). Published by Rosina Fasching, Klagenfurt 1983.

In 1987 the medical doctor and academically qualified biologist Dr. Reinhold Wiesner proved in a fields study that the biological food "Kombucha nach Dr. med. Sklenar" possesses a stunting effect on virosis that can stand comparison with the virustaticum "Helveferon" (= 12 different interferons).

Dr. Wiesner: "With the assistance of a bioresonator-test the potential difference of the biological food 'Kombucha nach Dr. med. Sklenar' was measured in millivolts as therapeutic energy dimension, possessing energy-supplying capacity for patients. This investigation was carried out with 246 chronically ill patients. Here Kombucha was given in combination with other remedies."

This comparison of measurement results between the biological food Kombucha and the clinically extensively tested Helveferon lead to the conclusion that **Kombucha builds up effectively the resistance in the sick body und puts in action the process of recovery of the body. Therefore Kombucha can be considered as a biological food of high value with virosis stunting effect, which does not produce any side effects or indigestibilities."**

Bio-electrical comparison of measurements between the biological food "KOMBUCHA nach Dr. med. Sklenar" (black) and the virustaticum Helveferon (grey).

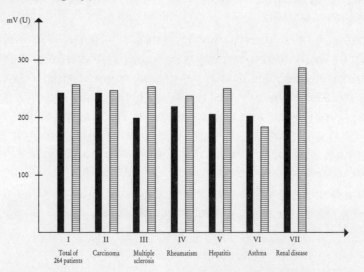

Source: Wiesner Laboratories, medical expertise about clinical experience in a practitioner's practice with the biological food "KOMBUCHA nach Dr. med. Sklenar and the virustaticum Helveferon, Schwanewede/FRG, 1987)"

Inevitably the question arises why a biological remedy with antibiotic properties should prove superior to chemotherapy, surgery and radiation treatment in cancer therapy and prophylaxis. To provide the right answer we have to go far back into the history of medicine.

Alongside academic medicine, which unfortunately does not uniformly back the theory of a cancer virus, researching physicians, bacteriologists and microbiologists have independently and repeatedly discovered parasitic micro-organisms in the tissue and blood of cancer patients, which are responsible for the development of a tumor.

As early as 1890 *Mr. Russel*, a Briton, described fuchsin particles inside the cancer cells. In 1898 *Sanfelice* pointed up the correlation of blastomyces with the development of cancer. A year later, *Josef Koch* found parasitic inclusions which he termed "Protozoon cancrosum" outside the cancer cells. In 1901 *Van Leyden* described the so-called "bird's eye cells" in cases of cancer. In 1902, *Borel* suspected a virus to be responsible for cancer triggered by parasites. A year later, the brothers *Otto* and *Wolfgang Schmidt* discovered vermicules and spores in cases of cancer. In 1904 *Doyen* reported on cocci and chains in tumorous tissue. In 1914 the bacteriologist *Mori* from Naples published his theory concerning the mycetic nature of an ultra-virus, whose transformation he had originally witnessed in 1910. In 1920 *Enderlein* discovered a micro-organism which can lead to cancer; he called it "Endobiont". In 1926 *Tissot* mentioned parasitic cancer elements as being amoeba-like forms. In 1928 *Heidenhain* (Tübingen) talked about a histologically traceable microbe in cancer. In 1932 *Von Neergaard* reported on the existence of blood parasites. In the same year *Von Brehmer* called cancer a virus disease and termed the responsible virus "Siphonospora polymorpha".[1] In December 1935 Von Brehmer's "Siphonospora polymorpha" was officially recognized as a new blood parasite by the Reichsgesundheitsamt (Ministry of Health) and by a commission of specially appointed clinicians and bacteriologists.[2]

The research findings of Dr. v. Brehmer culminated in the statement: "The cancer virus is the invisible stage of development of microscopic forms of 'Siphonospora polymorpha', which 'in vitro' can be made visible." In 1932 *Nebel* bred various growths from cancerous blood and

1 Besides the malaria plasmodia, 'Siphonospora polymorpha' is the only parasite attacking the red blood corpuscles, developing inside them and destroying them. It is responsible for most secondary anemias.
2 Wilhelm von Brehmer, M. D.: Siphonospora polymorpha, published by Br. Linck, Haag / Amper.

tissues and talked about a virus which he termed "Onkomyxa neoformans". In 1933 *Dechow* pointed out a variety of aspergillus as a cancer-causing organism, and *Gruner* and *Glower* in Canada found "Cryptomyces pleomorpha" in cases of cancer. In 1948 *Franz Gerlach* published his monography "Krebs und obligater Pilzparasitismus" (Cancer and Obligatory Fungus-Parasitism) in Vienna. Moreover, Prof. Gerlach reported from Africa that even uncivilized communities suffered from incredibly serious cases of cancer: in other words, cancer is not an affliction solely restricted to civilization! In 1951 *Lea Del Bo Rossi* in Milan published micro-photographs of the tiniest species of fungi found in cancer. In 1955 *Villequez* in Paris spoke about latent parasitism in blood cells. In 1956 *Scheller* published case histories of microscopy in the dark field: "Von Viren, Mitochondrien und vom Krebs" (On Viruses, Mitochondria and Cancer). In 1957 Prof. *Stanley* of Berkely University talked about the 'correlation between viruses and cancer'. In 1958 *Clara Fonti* from Milan published her "Aetiopathogenese des Krebses". (Aetiopathogenesis of Cancer), asserting the theory of cancer parasites with all its consequences. Likewise, *Schilling* succeeded in triggering tumors in mice by means of 'Siphonospora' rods. In the early 1970s *Prof. Gerhard Sauer* from the German Cancer Research Institute in Heidelberg stated in an article[1] named "Viruses as Accomplices, Cancer Research on New Paths" that after years of research he and his collaborators had succeeded in proving that viruses play a vital role in triggering tumors. In this case various types of papilloma viruses are involved; they are papova viruses, which are among the tiniest varieties. Last but not least, *R. Sklenar* with his blood picture proved that there are four stages of development of the blood parasite within the red blood corpuscles in precancerous and cancerous cases. In 1981 *Weber* from Erding/West Germany cultivated isolated cancer protozoa on freshly fertilized chicken eggs. Moreover he displayed micro-parasites and their various forms of development by means of an electronic camera and a TV screen. In 1981, after animal experiments at the University of Massachusetts in Worcester, *Mordes* and *Rossi* pointed out a substance circulating through the organism as the cancer-causing agent. When they linked up the blood circulation of tumor-free rats in parabiosis with animals suffering from cancer, they noted that tumors were triggered.[2]

1 Bild der Wissenschaft, Issue Feb. 1973.
2 Mordes, J. P. and Rossini, A. A. in "Science", Volume 213, p. 565

In 1984 the three virologists *Bishop, Vormus* (San Franzisco) and *Gallo* (Bethesda, Maryland) as well as the physicist *Rosenberg* (East Lansing, Michigan) were able to trigger cancer by means of the virus with apes.[1] – This list is far from being complete; countless other cancer researchers have come across micro-parasitism and have given the virus various names. What all these "discoverers" have in common is that they have found one and the same micro-organism and that official academic medicine has rejected them as outcasts. Even though an increasing number of cancer researchers throughout the world have come across viruses in cases of cancer, the virus theory is as yet far from being accepted; nor is the current cancer therapy based on the acceptance of a causative virus. No wonder that death rates from cancer remain frighteningly high und the diagnosis of "cancer" equals a death sentence. To be sure: only a correct and timely diagnosis makes a correct and timely therapy possible!

As a precondition for unterstanding the essential problematic nature of cancer as well as the divergent theses put forth by medical doctors, we have to deal with the research of *Prof. Dr. Günther Enderlein* concerning the nature of biological uniformity.[2]

In 1920 Enderlein discovered a micro-organism which can trigger cancer and called it "Endobiont". "Endobiosis" is the whole cyclogenesis, i. e. the processes of development of the fungus "Mucor racemosus Fresen", from primitive stages via bacterial stages to its culminating fungal stage. Obviously, micro-organisms have a biological variability. This is called pleomorphism or polymorphism. By simple breeding, any clever schoolboy can prove pleomorphism and the ascending development of *primitive stage – bacterium – fungus* of one and the same microorganism. The most primitive form of development of a microbe is the protite. It measures one hundred-thousandth of a millimeter and constitutes the original form of life itself – i. e. by no means a cell! Such a living, unassimilated protein colloid grows into a symprotite ball, also called mychite. This in turn grows into a mych and develops into a polyvalent nucleus called symmychon or cystite. When its nuclei divide, thecite comes into being, constituting the original form of a bacterial cell. It becomes visible by a microscopic enlargement of 20.000:1. Bacterial reproduction can result from simple division as well as sexually.

1 "Ärztliche Praxis" of Sep. 8, 1984, p. 1980.
2 Prof. Dr. Enderlein, Günther: Akmon, Volume I, Issues 1 and 2. Published by Ibica in 1955 and 1957, Aumühle/Hamburg. Also Volume I, Issue 3, published in 1959.

Bacterial cyclogenesis is the cycle of morphological development involving countless generations, from morphological uniformity (mychite) to morphological culmination, and again to morphological uniformity. The chronic complex of development of "endobiosis" is to be found among all mammals including man.

The culmination point of endobiontic cyclogenesis, i. e. the highest point of development of parasites, is to be found in its fungal stage. All previous stages including the initial phases of the fungal stage pose no danger to man, but as a consequence of further development catstrophic consequences such as cancer tend to ensue. All chronic diseases including cancer are by no means infectious diseases in the traditional sense, because an infection is inconsequential. All cells, including sperm and egg cells, all organs and tissues are infested by microscopic, invisible or barely visible primitive forms of "Endobiont".

Generally speaking, the "Endobiont" is the one noxious micro-organism with the greatest resistance against all kinds of exterior influences. It can survive – only in a dry state, however – *temperatures up to 590° F (310° C)* ...

> *Prof. Dr. Zettner:* "Dry protein is able to survive a temperature of 310° C with is germinating ability intact ..."[1]

In 1985 an American undersea-research expedition discovered a volcanic spring on the Pacific ocean floor, some 300 miles west of Seattle, at a depth of 7,900 feet. Despite a water temperature of 750° F (400° C) there were living organisms such as tube worms, giant shell-fish and bacteria.

... as well as extreme cold; it is immune to all chemotherapy and radiation therapy, because its resistance surpasses the resistance of the human body by far. *Budde-Grawitz* (Argentina) even managed to revive it from Egyptian mummies 10,000 years old. Also A. Cockburn and his research team from Detroit succeeded in proving intact proteins in Mummy "PUM II" from the Ptolemeic Era. And even Enderlein managed to cultivate the light brown spores of "Mucor racemosus Fresen" on a large scale from ancient sarcophagi in the catacombs near Rome. Note: After death human proteins, too, are absorbed by "Endobiont" and gradually transformed into spores of "Mucor racemosus Fresen".

---

1 The genetic importance of this peculiar quality of living colloidal proteins is based on an adaptation to purely biological conditions and an adaptation at the creation of the earth.

As a result, this parasite has never been conquered by conventional therapy methods! But:

It is one of the basic truths in biology, even a truism, that primitive bacteria dependent on an alkaline environment and fungi of all kinds dependent on an acidic environment, integrated on an agar plate, disturb each other's development and prevent each other's growth! In other words: The cyclogenetic development of the micro-organism cannot be enhanced by increased acidity of its nutritional base; on the other hand, it can be arrested (pH-level of the blood; acidity-alkaline balance of the human blood).

Based on his comprehensive and experimentally proven research work, Enderlein reaches the logical conclusion that the mystery of cancer can only be solved by biologists, because

living organisms can be combated by live matter only!

As *Dr. Sklenar* was able to note in decades of medical practice, every chronic disease including cancer is preceded by a general ailment of the organism, resulting mainly from a metabolic malfunction. This triggers an increasing accumulation of waste material in the body and creates the ideal environment where a virus can develop – but not necessarily does! In light of these facts it is not surprising, as a common saying goes, that "no cancer patient has a healthy digestive tract!"

Digestion is one of the decisive factors concerning health and illness. The complexity of metabolism determines our physical condition. Various producers of laxatives like to make use of true sayings of naturopaths, such as "Death lurks in your intestines!" On the one hand they are quite right in saying so, but on the other hand their various purgative teas and other laxatives fail to eliminate the root cause. It is not the symptom that ought to be treated, but the root cause of the digestive malfunction should be eliminated. Choosing the alternative of frugal and natural nutrition is inadequate, because not only our adulterated food, but also medical therapy involving antibiotics and radiation damage or, in extreme cases, kill the physiological intestinal bacteria in the colon. Who can boast of never having been given a chemical pill or penicillin? Antibiotics exert a negative influence on intestinal bacteria regardless of their composition or dosage, and as yet pharmacology has not been able to come up with a remedy to suppress the noxious bacteria while being harmless for physiologically essential bacteria.

The physiological phyla of bacteria (Escherichia coli) are not 'causative organisms', but vital agents of metabolism and defensive reactions (immune system). Cancer can be influenced via intestinal bacteria. Unfortunately doctors – after prescribing antibiotics – usually fail to repair the damage done to intestinal bacteria by means of colicines.

Since physiologically essential intestinal bacteria – especially the intestinal bacterium "Escherichia coli" – plays a part as vital for the well-being of the human body as a body organ[1], I will deal with their functions and tasks at greater detail:

- The substances of the vitamin-B group do not have to be consumed along with our food on a large scale, because intestinal bacteria produce them in large quantities and thus supply them to the organism in adequate amounts.
- Vitamin synthesis (processing and resorption) in man takes place mainly in the colon; it is the work of intestinal bacteria.
- The fermentative splitting of heavy or indigestible carbohydrates (starch, pectins, cellulose and cell fibers of plants) as well as proteins, especially those enclosed in plant cells; this function of coli bacteria is vital for herbivores.
- The antagonistic overgrowth and stifling of pathogenic bacteria: In this way coli bacteria form antibiotically active, protein-like colicines.
- The reduction of bilirubin in urobilin by intestinal bacteria does not occur when they are weakened, so the stool contains only bilirubin.
- Intestinal bacteria live in immune-biologically balanced symbiosis, i.e. there is an immune-biological interaction between the organism and the intestinal bacteria. In the mucous membranes of the intestines the bacteria keep up a constant reciprocal metabolism among one another. Disturbing these bacteria triggers various diseases.
- When the intestinal bacteria are weakened (non-physiological, but not yet pathological condition) the chemical and biological balance of the body suffers grave disturbances, dehydration and alterations of the electrolytic balance; it can even prevent the formation of antibodies against various viruses and their metabolic products.

1 See Prof. Dr. med. Ulrich Schneeweiß: Spezielle Microbiologie. Leitsätze für Studierende und Ärzte, Berlin, 1968, p. 54: "The physiological intestinal flora has vital responsibilitien in the life of the human being and the warm-blooded animal"

- Vitamin K 1 is produced physiologically by the intestinal bacteria; it is necessary for prothrombin synthesis in the mitochondria of the liver. When the vitamin-K synthesis is disturbed, the secondary consequence is that blood coagulation is hampered.
- Up to now the anti-carcinogetic vitamin K 2 has been found in coli bacteria only. With this intestinal bacterium (Escherichia coli) two kinds of asparagines have been found: The one enzyme was completely ineffectual against cancer, the other one a real hit. It displays the most effective tumor-arresting qualities observed up to now. To be sure, the asparagine used by cancer research today comes from these coli bacteria.
- Healthy intestinal bacteria dissolve various toxins which the liver can no longer handle. Thus liver and intestines are in constant interaction.
- 70 to 80 % of all defense cells (immune organs) are located in the intestinal wall. In order to function properly against viruses they need contact with healthy intestinal bacteria.

Combating cancer and countless other metabolic diseases is therefore correlated to stabilizing the intestinal bacteria.

Prof. Dr. Nissle was one of the first to describe the after-effects of a socalled "dysbacterium" of intestinal bacteria in the colon, and he developed an excellent coli compound[1] for curing and stabilizing the intestinal bacteria in the colon, both unphysiological and pathological. Dysbacterium is defined as the degeneration of the intestinal bacteria, which results in physical disturbances of all kinds. The toxins emanating from degenerated intestinal bacteria cause digestive ailments, afflictions in the liver-gall area, migraine, halitosis, rheumatic diseases, asthma, multiple sclerosis, eczema and cancer, to name just the most important ones.

---

1 "Mutaflor" (Mutation of intestinal bacteria) according to Prof. Dr. Nissle is a product of Ardeypharm Heilmittelgesmbh, Herdecke, GFR.

Part III

Treatment of Cancer and other Metabolic Diseases according to the Method of Dr. med. Sklenar

The treatment should be started by removing all focuses of disease (in the teeth, gallbladder, prostate, etc.). Dr. Sklenar achieved the best therapeutic success by combining TEA FUNGUS KOMBUCHA – COLICINES (Mutaflor, Colibiogen ampules, Colivit drinking ampules, Symbioflor II) with the oxygen activating gelum oral-rd[1].

The Treatment of Precancerosis (Cancer in its Preliminary Stages):

1. BEVERAGE OF KOMBUCHA: 3 x $^1/_4$ l per day

2. MUTAFLOR: (red capsules for adults) 1st to 5th day 1 capsule 1 hour before breakfast; from the 6th day on always 2 capsules. (Patients suffering from gastro-intestinal complaints should start with the yellow capsules).

The treatment of diagnosed cancer:

1. BEVERAGE OF KOMBUCHA: Up to 1 litre per day

2. KOMBUCHA CONCENTRATE: 3 x per day 1 teaspoon (ca. 15 drops) in 1 glass of water

3. MUTAFLOR: as above

4. GELUM ORAL-RD: 3 x per day 10 to 15 drops in 1 glass of water.

5. COLIBIOGEN AMPULES: 2 to 3 x per week 1 ampule; 3 x per year one cure with 18 ampules each.

Take all of these remedies for a period of two years and repeat the cures, if necessary.

---

1 See Dr. med. Rudolf Sklenar in: Sonderdruck aus Erfahrensheilkunde. Zeitschrift für die tägliche Praxis. Volume XIII. Issue 3. Karl F. Haug Verlag, Ulm/Donau 1964.

Part IV

Iris Diagnostics

Buried under a mountain of fanaticism, feeble-mindedness and mysticism on the one hand, and an unfounded aversion on the other, there lies the simple truth of iris diagnostics. As early as 1,000 B.C. man had noticed that whatever acted upon the human organism was not without effect upon the eye. By means of a magnifying glass the competent iris diagnostician sees various marks and phenotypes which go hand in hand with organic diseases.

Understanding iris diagnostics means collecting pieces of a mosaic, with the main object being observing rather than seeing. The main difficulty is understanding correlations in order to explain natural processes inside the body. Even though iridology's theoretical foundations are still unclear and mystic, extensive research comparing diagnostic results of clinicians to the ones of eye diagnosticians has shown beyond all doubt that there are correlations between iris marks and malfunctioning organs. To be sure, an eye diagnostician can only localize the affliction of an organ, but he cannot diagnose the nature of this affliction. Even in cases of acute organ malfunctions iris diagnostics will fail, but with chronic diseases iris marks will rarely be missing. In other words: at an early stage iris diagnostics can diagnose or, better, forecast a lingering disease which may break out years or even decades later as a metabolic disease.

The Hippocratic doctors of ancient Europe as well as, later on, Paracelsus, were accused of proceeding in a *prognostic* rather than a *diagnostic* way, because in their therapies they shunned the incurable. In other words, they did not wait for the disease to reach a fatal stage, but endeavored to realize at an early date *what would end badly.*

Iris diagnostics also makes possible an early prognosis. A disease is diagnosed before it causes pain, i. e. during its initial phase; for this reason it can be treated with considerably simpler, slighter and milder remedies than a later, painful stage.

In iris diagnostics *Dr. Sklenar* found invaluable criteria for recognizing lingering malignant processes at their earliest stages. He noted that changes inside the iris mainly affected the "iris ruffle", which allows conclusions concerning the intestines (colon). Patients suffering from circumscribed diseases, metabolic disturbances and cancer have irises marked by pigmentation consisting of brownish to black deposits. In many cases broad bands of pigmentation ringing the iris ruffle can be observed, sometimes cigar-shaped forms (torpedoes), which are surrounded by microscopic granular pigments. Years of research convinced Dr. Sklenar that from this pigmentation one can draw conclusions concerning a general malfunction of the human body. The cause can be found in the existence of a nidus (focal disease). There was always some conformity between pathological changes of the iris and the blood picture in Dr. Sklenar's examinations.

Nevertheless, iris diagnostics has not remained completely neglected by other doctors. *Dr.-Ing. V. Miszalok, M. D.* from the eye clinic of the Free University of Berlin, together with *Th. Seiler, M. D.,* and *Prof. J. Wollensak, M. D.*, developed a method for the early diagnosis of latent diseases by means of a precise, special camera. The photographs of the eyeground disclose immediately heretofore undiagnosed serious afflictions such as brain tumors, high blood pressure, arteriosclerosis and diabetes. Above all, this method allows arteriosclerosis to be diagnosed at such an early date that risks like cardiac infarction, stroke and thrombangiitis obliterans (smoker's leg) can be diagnosed and treated at an early stage.

There is no optically accessible part of the human organism with informative qualities comparable to the eyeground (fundus). In a healthy person it has a constantly uniform structure. But even the tiniest alteration spells alarm. At this stage other tests and diagnostic methods still tend to be 'negative'. Therefore it is advisable to have an annual "eye photograph" taken and compared to the one from the previous year: this would give an indication of a person's physical condition. Dr. Miszalok is optimistic: "In ten years' time, every prophylactic examination will start out with an examination of the eyeground."

What somebody without a special camera might erroneously interpret as a "personal peculiarity" in his eye — like his unique finger print — is nothing less than a sign of a circumscribed disease, metabolic disturbance or an injury.

To be sure, the basic precondition for understanding and applying iris diagnostics is a universal attitude toward the human organism and its diseases.

Part V

Haemogram according to Dr. Sklenar

In the dyed blood smear *Dr. Sklenar* was able to prove the existence of viruses which are responsible for cancer. With his relatively simple and quick method of dyeing blood, precancerous (pretumorous) stages and cancer can be unequivocally diagnosed at an early time. After years of research he was able to find the four visible stages of the virus in its fungal phase.

The blood parasite attacks the red blood corpuscles (erythrocytes), develops inside them and destroys them. At the beginning only a few spores and slightly damaged erythrocytes can be seen. In precancerous stages, years before a tumor develops, granula (stage I) and thorn-apple forms (stage II) can be seen. In the course of the disease the thorn-apple forms multiply considerably, and finally blisters develop (stage III).

At an advanced stage of the tumor the erythrocytes appear to be hollowed out from the inside, so that in the end only ring forms remain (stage IV). Also the existence of megalocytes points to a malignant stage.

Moreover, in precancerous stages the patients feel ill; they will consult specialists and clinics, but the diagnosis is still 'negative'. It has been noted that during these pretumorous stages the iris and the blood picture are distinctly 'positive' and display the same changes as the diagnosed cases of cancer (tumors). Here the same therapy is successful.

All stages of Sklenar's blood picture must be intensively treated with the Kombucha drink, Kombucha-D 1 drops, colicines and a compound for increasing oxygen in the body tissue (gelum oral rd). This is necessary because, as *Dr. v. Brehmer* was able to note, mental stress such as depression, shock, sorrow, anguish, fear etc. shifts the pH-level of the blood toward the alkaline side and thus aids the virus in its development.

After an average four to six weeks the above-mentioned therapy will normalize the blood count, eliminate the deposits in the iris and increase the patient's well-being.

Blood Dyeing according to Dr. Sklenar

1. Blood smear to be well air-dried (at least 30 minutes)
2. Fix: 3 minutes in pure alcohol
3. Air-dry (at least 10 minutes)
4. Dye blue: 2 minutes
5. Rinse with Aqu. bidest.
6. Dye red: 3 minutes
7. Rinse with Aqu. bidest.
8. Air-dry

The examination occurs in the light field by means of oil immersion. The blood is examined only in well-dyed places, and only where the corpuscles can be seen individually.

Even new implements should be cleaned before use.

Part VI

Reports on Therapeutic Success

Cases from the Medical Practice

When treating intensively with "Kombucha nach Dr. Sklenar" and with colicines, the haemogram normalizes within the next four to six months, the sediments in the iris disappear and the patient feels better.

Some Remarkable Cases from Dr. Sklenar's Practice:[1]

"Mrs. D., born 1941, came to see me in a desolate state on 18 August 1982. In February 1981 the patient had a uterectomy. A few months later sarcomata of the bone were removed from her left forearm. Some time later her left armpit was curetted. The patient was hospitalized in clinics and also in the "Tumorzentrum Essen". She was extremely depressive, had thoughts of suicide and was most of the time confined to bed."

During her examination on 18 August 1982 it was noted that the iris was surrounded by a dark ring of pigments.

The signs of the lower abdominal region were discernable. The haematogram was characterized by masses of vesicles. I prescribed her the following:

2 x per day 1 wine glass of Kombucha; 1 x per day 2 capsules Mutaflor; 3 x per day 15 drops of Kombucha D 1; 3 x per day 10 drops Gelum oral-rd for oxygenization of the tissue.

Already after one week of therapy her feeble condition disappeared and the patient was less confined to the bed. The reexamination on 22nd November of this year showed **a clarification of the pigments in the iris and her haemogram was normal! Her state of health was normal.** The patient could work again, was full of joy and of optimism.

1 Letter of Dr. R. Sklenar dated December 1982 to the headquarters of "Gesamtprogramm zur Krebsbekämpfung" in Bonn.

EYE MELANOMA

Mrs. G. M., born 1904, has been suffering from asthma emphysema and glaucoma since 1948. In August 1971 a melanoma of the choroid was discovered in the right eye. The patient should be operated immediately, but she refused it. After she was informed she left the hospital on her own responsibility.

When I examined her I found in her iris clear signs of cancer and masses of vesicles in the blood. The treatment that was immediately started with the usual remedies (Kombucha, Mutaflor, Colibiogen ampules) soon brought the desired recuperation. Four months later the signs of cancer disappeared.

During an examination on 17 September 1980, once again many pigments were discovered in the iris and strongly positive values in the blood. Patient admitted that the tea fungus had died and that she also had stopped taking 'the expensive red capsules' (Mutaflor) for quite some time. An energetic therapy was started immediately and it brought normal results after six months. In serious cases constant control and therapy are necessary.

In 1982 – the patient was **treated without interruption – normal results were achieved**. The patient feels physically and mentally well, and she does not need assistance. For 15 years already she has been taking Glukat-Komplex drops (Spemann) against her troubles of glaucoma.

Two sisters of the patient had perished miserably of cancer.

TUMOUR OF THE THYROID GLAND

Mr. H. E., born 1933, pharmaceuticals representative, has come to see me for 15 years. On 19 June 1980 he asked me to examine him. He indicated that he has had medical treatment from a specialist for the past three years and got hormone preparations for the thyroid gland. He has a medical examination semiannually.

In the meantime the diagnosed tumour of the thyroid gland grew to the size of an egg. When I examined him his iris and his blood were positive. Since August 1980 the patient has been taking regularly every day two big glasses full of Kombucha; he did not take Mutaflor. In March 1981 the specialist re-examined the patient. **By that time the tumour had been reduced by two thirds! The iris and the blood tests were nearly normal.** The patient had no more complaints.

TUMOUR OF THE BRAIN

By A. F., born 1924, a tumour of the brain was discovered in a hospital in April 1974. After the patient had been informed about the risks of an operation he refused the operation.

On 18 April 1974 I examined the patient. The left iris was surrounded by a ring of pigments. In the section of the brain there were deep lines and a big, macroscopical, black pigmental mole. The lines were covered with macroscopical pigments.

The patients received 18 injections of Colibiogen and drank two wine glasses of Kombucha per day. After some weeks the complaints were reduced. In the clinic they ascertained that the tumour had decreased in size and some time later that **the tumour had disappeared entirely. The iris pigments had disappeared completely, the black pigmental mole had turned lighter.**

The patient was medically examined and treated in the ambulatory of the clinic. Iris and blood are normal. The patient feels well.

SERIOUS DISEASE OF THE PELVIC ORGANS

Mrs. O. R., born 1922, had to undergo a radical operation in 1973. In 1979 again cancer formation in the vagina, she had 18 radiotherapies and got two temporary fillings containing radium. A partial resection of the vagina was carried out.

On 4 May 1981 Mrs. R. came to consult me. She was in a very desolate state of health. She had strong archorrhagia and therefore had to wear thick nappies. The iris indicated a serious metabolic disease. There were masses of sediments of uric acid and of cholesterol. Furthermore, there were large pigmentations (macr. and micr.) in the intestinal region. Moreover, there were uterus and vagina signs as well as an extensive ring of calcerous degenerations. The haemogram also showed serious alterations: It was full of ring-like forms. (The erys = red blood cells were degenerated to thin rings.) After giving the patient Mutaflor and Kombucha for six months, the patient has been restored to the extent that she is able to do her housework and to untertake short journeys. In the haemogram new formation of sound erys = red blood cells was recognizable. In the iris the **pigments became lighter and smaller. On 18 March 1982 the findings were normal.** The patient said she felt quite strong and even goes dancing. One of her sisters had a utereetomy.

GASTRO-INTESTINAL DISTURBANCES

Mrs. R. L., born 1937, suffered from a sort of feverish infection in December 1981 / January 1982. For three months she received a penicillin depot treatment. Her state of health aggravated visibly. She consulted several specialists, but the various medical examinations did not reveal anything. She consulted, on her own, several doctors and therapists, without any result. She then was referred to a psychiatrist. Since he could not ascertain any somatic changes he recommended autogenous training. It did not help. The patient wasted away, could not eat anything anymore.

On 17 May 1982 the patient went to consult me in this desolate state. The iris showed makr. and mikr. pigments of the intestine. The blood showed masses of vesicles in the erys. The patient was very agitated and nervous. I prescribed her drops of Kombucha, „Urtinktur" and Mutaflor. When reexamined on 13 June 1982 the patient was back to normal. She could eat and drink again and had put on weight. There were **hardly any signs in the iris, the haemogram showed normal results.**

On 2 July 1982 the patient said: "I feel well – how happy I am!"

LUNG TROUBLES

J. F., born 1957, underwent 6 years of medical treatment with a specialist. Her state of health aggravated constantly despite the many tablets she had to swallow every day. She suffered from fits of coughing and a severe constipation, that could not be relieved. She took already 15 laxatives per day, prescribed by the physician in charge!

In January 1982 the medical examination showed strong signs of the lung in the iris and severely affected bowels. The blood count was strongly positive: stages III and IV.

After taking Mutaflor and Kombucha for only three days the bowels were regular and the cough eased off. The patient has been drinking one litre of Kombucha per day. By the end of September 1982 the reexamination showed a **nearly normal haemogram and hardly any signs in the iris.**

The patient feels well and she felt "like a new person".

Reports on Therapeutic Success

The following statements were sent to Dr. Rudolf Sklenar or to the author unasked. They constitute – to show the variety and the extensive field of activity of Kombucha – only a selection of the innumerable amount of letters from several countries.

Mrs. B. from Baden:
"I would like to say the following about your wonderful tea fungus Kombucha. I am 65 years old and have been suffering from **terrible headache** for 35 years ... After taking Kombucha for three months I no longer suffer from headache. I am extremely happy, no one could help me, only pills. Now I do not need them any more."

Mr. G. from Stade:
"After a short time I noticed that this fungus can heal **gastritis**."

Mrs. T. from Waldmoor:
"I cannot describe my enthusiasm. When I was 30, now I am 45 years old, my hair turned grey. Now my natural **hair colour** comes back. I can hardly believe it. My **nails** are also stronger. My **allergy** has improved, my **skin** is not so dry anymore and my **joints** are no longer so stiff."

Mrs. R. from Würnsdorf:
"For 8 years I have been suffering from **gout** in the feet. Last year I started a Kombucha cure. I noticed a **strong dehydrating effect** and my complaints now are negligible. Before the cure I suffered from really strong pain and no other remedy could cure it constantly."

Mr. M. from Haarlem (medical doctor):
"After having (come to know) the fungus, I prescribed it with lots of success to **children suffering from bronchitis.**"

Mrs. A. from Villach:
"Before taking Kombucha regularly I had very **low blood pressure** which rose to the normal value within a few months (...). It also has a very positive effect on the **digestion** ... substantial **improvement of the blood count.** I also heard from several acquaintances that they feel very well."

Mr. K. from Villach:

"Because of **severe gout** I was able to move only with the help of a stick. After three months the state of health improved visibly, now I am without pain."

Mr. E. and Mrs. St. from Villach:

"... had a **high cholesterol level** that dropped, after a few months, to the normal level."

Mrs. L. from Villingen:

"... I tried the tea fungus Kombucha by myself. In the beginning I was much afraid because the **level of sugar** varied **between 280 and 400.** Furthermore I suffered from **water in the feet up to the knees,** that could not be cured even in a special clinic. Well, the time from July to the end of November I considered more or less as a trial period. 1) The main thing: the glucometabolism regulation test showed a decrease of the values to normal values of 105 to 108, the doctor was dumbfounded when he heard the news. 2) The water in the feet disappeared completely. What a wonderful success thanks to your product."

Mrs. R. from Würnsdorf:

"I am glad to tell you that Kombucha drops not only help to cure **gout,** but also my **intestinal troubles** have been reduced from the time I started to take them."

Mrs. L. from Graz:

"Since the operation of my intestine (cancer) in September 1981 I have been drinking the Kombucha beverage every day, and I believe it has helped me considerably. I feel well and do not suffer from any complaints ... My **rheumatic nodes** of which my fingers were strongly affected, have, in any case, decreased in size, although I do not take any medicine. It seems Kombucha has helped also here."

Mrs. R. from Gailitz:

"After having suffered for years from intestinal troubles – I **did not have defecation without laxatives** – I started to drink Kombucha. After half a year I no longer needed laxatives. My haemogram has also improved considerably."

Mrs. R. from Arnoldstein:
"In December 1983 I had to undergo a gynaecologic operation, because I had **carcinoma of the uterus.** After undergoing a radiation therapy, I was in a bad state of health, my **haemogram was bad** and I **suffered greatly from intestinal troubles.** Since I have been taking the Kombucha tea, I feel better every day, my blood count improved every week and the defecation has normalized. I feel well again and have recovered. I do not take any other medicine. I am completely healthy again as proved by my last medical examination in the hospital."

Mrs. St. from Ybbs:
"Last year my son had a serious car accident with grave head injuries. Since he was for a long time unconscious, and subsequently suffered from **serious lack of concentration** I gave him, to improve the supply of oxygen, Kombucha-D1-drops... His state of health improved to the extent that he could take up and continue his university studies. I did not even dare to think of that before."

Mrs. T. from Lavamünd:
"I had **cancer in its early stage** and was not only cured from this disease by taking Kombucha, but also feel more fit now and healthier than ten years ago."

Mrs. F. from Lavamünd:
"Every year in spring and in autumn I have been suffering from serious **gastro-intestinal complaints.** With the help of Kombucha combined with colicines I was able to heel my painful **gastritis** and have been without complaints for several years. Furthermore the **asthmatic troubles** my child suffered from have improved considerably."

Mr. Sch. from St. Veit/Glan:
"I have known Kombucha since the 1930ies and have been able to watch and to experience that Kombucha is a vitamin-rich home remedy that strengthens and refreshes the vital force."

Mrs. Sp. from Klagenfurt:
"My husband drinks Kombucha like brook water. Although he does not take any medicine he has had no more **attacks of the gout**."

Mr. W. from Lindenfels:

"The tea fungus Kombucha stirs up memories of my childhood. My mother was suffering from **diabetes** and she said that this liquid had a very good effect on diabetes."

Mrs. K. from Nohen:

"I used to suffer from *high blood pressure* and have a myoma. The blood pressure has come down to normal. The beverage of Kombucha does me good."

Mr. L. from Friesenried:

"The effect of the prepared tea is very often amazing. For example, my mother (73 years) got rid of her **rheumatic troubles** within only a few weeks. In addition the **pressure of the eye**, which has been **too high** for many years, has reduced to normal values, which astonished tremendously the oculist in charge. An **improvement of the sight** was the consequence."

Mr. L. from Haslach:

"I know a woman who had **stomach cancer** and was cured from it by Kombucha."

Mrs. D. from Velzen:

"For one year I have been taking regularly every day the recommended remedy and have put on 5 kilos of **weight**, that had been down to 48 kg, during the past two months."

Mrs. D. from Munich:

"I have been drinking the Kombucha tea for three weeks and I feel much better than before, fresher, younger and fitter (not so tired anymore because of **low blood pressure**)."

Mrs. H. from Senftenberg:

"I suffer a lot from **constipation** and since I have been drinking the tea it improves."

Mrs. J. from Gießen:

"Two years ago I had influenza. From that time on I have been suffering from **secretion of mucus from the throat.** The strong secretion was reduced tremendously after drinking Kombucha for only eight days."

Mrs. K. from Vienna:
"I have been drinking Kombucha already for one year. I would not want to miss this beverage! I am a bit sad that my family laughs at me and does not drink it. Since I have been taking it I feel well and my **intestinal complaints** – constant **strong flatulence,** no matter what I ate – have disappeared. Up to now I could not find anything bad about it, only agreeable things."

Mr. Sch. from Kimratshofen:
"I suffer from **Morbus Hodgkin St. III b** and get chemotherapy. For 2 $^1/_2$ months I have been drinking also the Kombucha tea, that does me very good."

A medical doctor from Kempten:
"I myself am a **dialysis patient.** Therefore I may drink only very little liquid and I drank Kombucha – without any great expectations – primarily because it is a thirst-quenching drink, you only need a few mouthfuls. We – the dialysis patients – need to have made a long series of laboratory analyses in longer intervals (about 8 to 10 weeks). Up to now it used to be normal that the values of creatinine and urea increased regularly, despite dialysis. To my great surprise the last check showed a considerable reduction of these values. For several weeks I have been taking Kombucha, but otherwise there was no change in my way of life, food, dialysis, medication."

A group of researchers from Marburg:
"We concern ourselves with orgone energy and the accumulation of atmospheric energy in practice. Since Wilhelm Reich made it public, it is known that bacteria from yoghurt cultures accumulate large quantities of orgone and transfer this energy with the help of bacteria to people who eat yoghurt. The natural remedy Kombucha also shows in its application an enormous improvement of the energy level for the user.

"Just one sentence from our ... publication after W. Reich: **In the proximity of blood cells that are strongly charged with orgone energy not pathogenic organisms can exist.**"

"The importance of using Kombucha in all households is well known to you."

Mrs. N. from Launsdorf:

"Since some of my acquaintances convinced me about the wholesome effects of this beverage I have nearly become addicted to it. I rise every day at 5 o'clock and can hardly wait for this moment when I take the glass with Kombucha. For the past 10 to 15 years I have been suffering from terrible **pain in the left upper half of my breast,** no doctor could find anything so that I **felt like a person who fancies herself ill ... Every blood test showed an elevated blood sedimentation.**

Since my **gallbladder was removed,** a doctor said that it might be the formation of the scar that gives me this feeling of an inflammation. But I have a different opinion, because, since I have been drinking Kombucha, the pain has nearly disappeared completely. But if I stop taking this beverage, because I ran out of it, the inflammation comes back quite easily."

Mrs. K. from Höxter:

"I suffer from strong arthrosis and I am very pleased with the result. I no longer need medicaments (against rheumatism)."

KOMBUCHA for the healthy person

People often call the tea fungus Kombucha a vitality strengthening luxury food that increases wellbeing, and one likes to drink it, because of its good taste or simply as a thirst-quenching beverage. Many people regard this beverage as an excellent preventive and observe a reduced susceptibility to colds."

Kombucha is very popular with competitive athletes and spare time sportsmen, who prefer a reasonable form of nutrition and enrich their nourishment with appropriate dietary means. It is not by accident that Kombucha has become known among sportsmen as making fit.

As already mentioned in Part I, teeth can be protected notably against caries, if Kombucha is taken regularly.

For some definitely healthy people Kombucha is simply a "tranquilizer". When thinking of the extent on environmental pollution and its burden on the human being, on his immune system and his detoxication centre, it reassures many of them to have at hand a powerful remedy for the purification of the body.

Other people make once a year a cure with the Kombucha beverage, just like they give their car annual service.

A Well-known Household Beverage

"The tea fungus Kombucha thrives in our vicinity and enjoys great popularity. I must continually brew vast quantities of it. Recently I was told by a clergyman (born in 1907) that during his childhood in Pommern he was given this beverage every day when he came home from school." *(15)*

"I've known about the Kombucha beverage and the fungus since 1925. My lay practitioner, who has been treating me for years, was personally presented with the fungus in 1980 by Dr. Sklenar himself." *(18)*

"I've known about the fungus since my youth but up until now, when I've grown old, I've not been able to learn more about it. My aunt kept it handy, and we children always rejoiced when we were given a glassful. Then she died and we got no more of it. Now I'm very interested in this fungus." (22)

"I'm 72 years old and I remember that during my childhood my mother also had the tea fungus, But as she possessed no written information about it, she was surely not clear about its significance in human health. Then the fungus was lost when our house was remodeled in 1928." *(39)*

"The reason I value the Kombucha fungus so highly is because my deceased mother prepared it herself. Back then I was just a young girl, and it had always tasted so good to us. Unfortunately I can no longer ask my mother about it (she was 90 years old)." *(43)*

"I read your book about the Kombucha tea fungus with great interest, and recalled that at my aunt's in East Prussia we children found this beverage very refreshing. She kept the fungus in a stoneware crock, and it was replenished time and again." *(44)*

"In my childhood many years ago my dear mother made it often, as I still can well remember. But during the war, or perhaps even earlier, we stopped drinking it, and never heard about it again." *(45)*

"I'm very interested in the Kombucha fungus, which my grandmother called 'Schombuggo'." *(46)*

"Even today I can still remember that tasty beverage. During my school days we always had that fungus in my grandmother's house. But during the war – I also had to flee from Czechoslovakia – the fungus was lost to us." *(72)*

"In the thirties, on occasional visits to my grandmother in Linz, it was always a special attraction for us children when our grandmother served us a glass of "Tschambuco". We would gladly take up this old practice again in order to avoid drinking the products of the beverage industry." *(73)*

"My father has known about Kombucha since his childhood, when the tea fungus was almost a fad-beverage in Munich." *(75)*

"In 1930 my mother was already preparing the fungus for us children, and we drank it with great enjoyment." *(93)*

"In my family the tea fungus was a daily drink until 1944. In that year we were bombed out, and naturally the tea-fungus days were over. After the war I endeavored futilely to find it again. My joy is that much greater when I read about it now." *(94)*

"My parents already knew about this fungus in the thirties, and were always quite enthusiastic." *(118)*

"My mother had this tea fungus in the thirties. I'm 74 years old, and have been searching for the fungus for decades!" *(119)*

"I've known about Kombucha since the thirties, and could time and again observe and experience that Kombucha is a vitamin-rich, vitality-strengthening and refreshing household staple." *(185)*

"In general practice we concern ourselves with orgone energy, and with gathering energy from the atmosphere. Through Wilhelm Reich it has long been known that yogurt-cultured bacteria store large a mounts of orgone, and that this energy is transferred to yogurt eaters by way of the bacteria. The natural remedy Kombucha likewise manifests in its effects an enormous energy increase in its users. Just one sentence from our work according to Wilhelm Reich: No pathogenic organism can exist in the vicinity of blood cells abundantly charged with orgone. You sure know how vital it is to introduce Kombucha into every household." *(186)*

Miscellaneous Complaints

"My husband and I have been drinking Kombucha daily for about half a year. I learned about it from a friend. We drink it gladly and it gives us a feeling of well-being. Since then I've been able to manage more; I'm no longer so hectic and I'm better poised."

"In our circle of friends Kombucha has effected much relief in the areas of high blood pressure, hip-joint pain, and digestive disorders." *(61)*

"We had a Kombucha fungus for four years, which we unfortunately lost due to low temperatures. We were so sorry because the tea had done so well by us. Since then my mother's eyes and her circulation have gotten worse. Where can I obtain a tea fungus again?" *(64)*

"I've been preparing the tea fungus according to your directions for some months now. I've bought several copies of your book and presented them to friends and relatives."

"Meanwhile we've gained some experience with the fungus and the tea made from it. The effect of the prepared tea is often astonishing. For example, within a few weeks my mother's rheumatic discomfort abated. Likewise, to the amazement of the opthalmologist treating her, her intra-ocular pressure, too high for many years, subsided to normal values. That was and is coupled with an improvement in visual faculties." *(82)*

"It's beneficial for one to drink this Kombucha beverage. I've been taking it for a very long time, I believe. The initial effect was felt as it went through and through my body. Shooting pains on my cranium are no longer there. Another thing: My nervous system has become quite placid, and also my mood in general." *(83)*

"I've purchased the Kombucha tea fungus and am quite surprised at the number of ailments it alleviates." *(113)*

"My husband and I have been drinking Kombucha tea for six months. It agrees with me very well; – my stomach and bowels have greatly improved. I also take Mutaflor. I must add that I've been having trouble with my stomach and digestion for some 30 years; without cathartics my digestive processes would have been completely blocked. Now I'm able to have a bowel movement every second day, and for that I'm very grateful. I scarcely need take anything for my stomach either."
"Aside from all that, my hair has become darker." *(126)*

"I can't describe my astonishment. I'm 45 years old today, but at 30 my hair turned almost totally grey. Now I'm suddenly getting my hair color back; I can hardly believe it. My fingernails have become harder, too. My allergic condition has improved, my skin is no longer so dry, and my joints are not as stiff as before. All in all, an amazing improvement in my state of health." *(162)*

"Year after year, in spring and fall, serious stomach and bowel disturbances used to set in. Then with Kombucha and colic preparations I was able to heal my gastric ailments and have been for some years completely distress-free. Moreover, my child's asthma trouble has improved substantially." *(178)*

"I (52 years old) have been drinking the Kombucha beverage for about four months, and it's been amazingly good for me. My nervous state of exhaustion and my feelings of anxiety, from which I've been suffering for thirty years, are not nearly as acute as they were. I had never thought that even Kombucha could have an effect on such disorders." *(67)*

"I've been suffering from depression for 13 years. I often had such anxiety and uneasiness. Five months ago I started to drink Kombucha tea from the health food store. Then things started to change with me, and after four weeks my state of health began to improve. The anxiety and uneasiness disappeared. It went well with me and I was able to reduce the dosage of Lexotamil tablets I'd been taking. As I only have a small pension, I cut my Kombucha to one glass per day. Then things got worse with me, anxiety and uneasiness returned; indeed not as severe, but I've again lost the courage to face life. I've resumed taking the Ω tablets that I'd set aside. I also suffer from rheumatism, although that's improved somewhat. I still have acute headache attacks, but I sleep a little better. Please, I'm asking for your advice." *(138)*

Arthrosis

"The taking of twelve liters of Kombucha has been very good for my arthrosis. My sister's circulatory disorders have also disappeared after taking a like amount." *(6)*

"It's been ten years since I started taking the fungus, and I''m very happy with it. I continually recommend this beverage to other people, for I'm convinced of its great remedial effects. I suffer from severe arthrosis, and am quite satisfied with the tea's success; I require no other medication (rheumatism remedies)." *(95)*

Breathing difficulty, Bronchitis

"I've been drinking about a half-liter Kombucha almost daily for the past four weeks, and have less and less problems with my chronic respiratory tract dysfunction. Therefore I'm very enthusiastic." *(111)*

"Every morning I've drunk a glass of Kombucha on an empty stomach; my metabolic dysfunction has regressed. My catarrhal discharge has lessened and my bronchitis has improved." *(51)*

"I am a doctor. Since I've become acquainted with the fungus, I prescribe it for bronchitis-afflicted children with great success." *(166)*

Enthusiasm

"I've owned a Kombucha fungus for a good year, and my circle of Kombucha-drinking friends and acquaintances has grown considerably during this time.

None of us would ever give it up, and we perform the ritual of Kombucha preparation weekly." *(66)*

"Recently I read your book about the Kombucha fungus, and I'd like to prepare the tea myself as a preventive remedy. Several of my friends drink the tea regularly, and are enthusiastic." *(102)*

"During our vacation I put my fungus in someone else's care and didn't have the heart to take it back, as the beverage worked so well with the family I'd lent it to. My husband, my children and I are also just as enthusiastic about Kombucha. Please send me another tea fungus for ourselves." *(137)*

Blood Pressure

"We obtained a Kombucha fungus from friends one year ago. They had had beneficial experiences with it and were of the opinion that we should also give it a try. That we did! I mean, since then everything goes much better, especially with me. My disorders caused by low blood pressure have completely disappeared." *(20)*

"I'm enthusiastic about Kombucha tea. I suffered from unexplainably-high blood pressure, which condition markedly improved in a really short while, so much so that I could stop taking other medicines. My skeptical doctor was amazed (still doesn't believe it)." *(74)*

"I had been drinking Kombucha tea daily for fifteen months, and it gave me a feeling of well-being. My blood sugar level was good, my blood pressure re-stabilized, and as I said, I felt well all-around.

I've drunk no more Kombucha for the past four weeks, and consequently I'm feeling worse. The fungus I had been using seems to have died and no longer regenerates itself." *(98)*

"My wife has been drinking Kombucha tea for some time, tea which she herself prepares; in her opinion she hasn't felt so well for a long while. Her ailments, such as pain in her legs and low blood pressure, have markedly improved." *(139)*

"I had very low blood pressure before I started taking Kombucha regularly; after several months it has increased to normal values. Further- more it's had a positive influence on digestion, and . . . a considerable improvement in blood-count." *(167)*

"I suffered from high blood pressure, and also had a myoma. My blood pressure has become normal again. The Kombucha beverage agrees with me exceptionally well." *(180)*

Cholesterol

"I began to drink Kombucha tea about one year ago. After a few weeks my cholesterol level decreased to 195. I ceased drinking it because of an illness (actually, a heart operation), but have now resumed the tea cure as of a couple of weeks ago with the hope that my cholesterol level (now 253!) will again be reduced." *(49)*

"I obtained the tea fungus Kombucha a scant year ago, and at irregular intervals have been taking tea I myself prepared. I've ascertained that it has helped me, and attribute the reduction in my slightly elevated cholesterol level to the tea's effect." *(86)*

"I got a Kombucha fungus about two years ago, before I even bought your book. It first took effect on my high cholesterol level, which not only ceased rising, but decreased from 329 to 279." *(105)*

"I always had too high a level of blood lipids, and much flatulence. I've been drinking Kombucha tea for about three months, and have just- had a new analysis. It's only 199 – I'm utterly amazed. I hadn't been on a strict diet, and earlier when I was dieting the level didn't drop. Now it stays down with Kombucha without any special diet." *(121)*

"My interest in Kombucha fungus is especially great, mainly because my husband is ill with a cholesterol-induced metabolic dysfunction. May I tell you that several of my acquaintances have been able, by taking the fungus liquid, to bring their excessive cholesterol values down to normal levels without the aid of other medication." *(134)*

"As I've now been drinking Kombucha tea regularly for more than a year, I can pass this happy news on to you. My blood was just re-examined and my cholesterol level, which was until now markedly elevated, is now within a normal range." *(147)*

". . . both of us had a high cholesterol level, which sank to a normal value after a few months." *(169)*

Diabetes

"I am a diabetic, and have been drinking Kombucha tea prepared with fruit sugar for a half year. Strip tests show that this tea I myself prepare is sugar-free after 10 days, that is, fully fermented. For this reason I believe that your assertion that Kombucha tea is not suitable for diabetics isn't strictly true." *(8)*

"I've been preparing the fungus tea for some time. I have advanced-age diabetes, and unfortunately ascertained that my diabetic value has increased. Thereupon I tried to prepare the tea using fruit sugar. It seems to work out better, although I of course don't know whether this is compatible with the tea fungus, nor whether it causes it to change." *(33)*

"My husband had high blood pressure and diabetes. Both levels rose high above normal when he started to drink Kombucha. You know, we like drinking the tea, only not the black variety." *(34)*

"For the past two months I've been taking 1/8 liter of Kombucha after lunch each day. I feel very well, and the tea tastes good, but my blood sugar level doesn't decrease. I've been a diabetic for 15 years." *(71)*

"I obtained the Kombucha from a friend, and meanwhile I've also read your book. In this regard I have only one question: I'm a diabetic dependent on insulin, and have tried to prepare the tea with Siomon (trade name) or other dietetic sweeteners. Unfortunately it went bad after the second try. Indeed, one can't prepare it without sugar. Are there drops suitable for diabetics available?" *(128)*

"My wife suffers from diabetes. A colleague at work recommended Kombucha, saying that her diabetic parents had had some success with it. We've been drinking the tea regularly for three weeks. My wife took a blood-sugar test today; the results showed that it was more than 60 points higher than the previous test." *(156)*

"I've been regularly obtaining from an acquaintance Kombucha tea that she prepares herself. Taking it was beneficial in several ways, but for the second time recently it pointed to the fact that I have a case of creeping (gradually increasing) diabetes. The first time, through a strict diet and by giving up the Kombucha I got the condition under control. After a certain interval I started taking Kombucha again. Now, for the second time, my condition seems to be taking the same course." *(157)*

"I've been drinking Kombucha fungus tea for the past half-year, with very good results. Now, unfortunately, my doctor has let me know that my blood-sugar level has sharply increased. Now I'm wondering whether the tea fungus is to blame." *(158)*

"I've been a Kombucha fan for a short while. I've tried to prepare the tea with dietetic sugar, but of course it doesn't ferment." *(160)*

"I've been drinking Kombucha fungus tea for almost a year. I've felt very well, and have also lost a few pounds. One day my doctor informed me that my blood-sugar level has risen to more than 400. Naturally I immediately ceased drinking the tea and had to go on a strict diet. My levels are somewhat normal once again. Is the fungus tea unsuitable for diabetics?" *(159)*

"I have already heard and read very much about your Kombucha fungus tea. My family doctor said that I should give it a try. But as I am a diabetic, have stomach and liver disorders and abnormal bacterial flora, I can't tolerate the fungus tea prepared with common sugar. I have a constant excess of stomach acid, gastritis and duodenitis." *(161)*

"I tried out the Kombucha fungus myself. With great anxiety at the beginning, for my blood-sugar level ranged between 280 and 400.
Besides, I was suffering from excess water absorption in my feet and lower legs up to the knee, a condition even a special clinic couldn't relieve. Well, from July until the end of November is a good and sufficient period for a trial run. 1.) Mainly, my blood-sugar level sank to a normal value of 105 to 108; the doctor was amazed. 2.) The water in my lower extremities has completely disappeared. Aren't those wonderful results, thanks to your product?" *(170)*

Dialysis

"As a dialysis patient I am unfortunately condemned to the least possible liquid intake, and I drank Kombucha with no great or special expectations, mainly because it only took a few swallows to quench thirst. At fairly long intervals (some 8 to 10 weeks) we dialysis patients undergo an extensive series of laboratory tests. In spite of dialysis it was until now usual that the creatinin and urea values continuously increased. To my great surprise, at the last control session there was a considerable decrease in these values. I have been taking Kombucha for several weeks, but otherwise during this period nothing has changed in my living habits, food intake, dialysis or medication." *(183)*

Inflammation

"I'm so enthusiastic about Kombucha. It's also helpful to me as a gargle (I've had and have festering tonsils), as well as something to rub on inflamed places (my small child's soreness disappeared in one day; nothing else was successful in easing his teething)" *(63)*

"Together with several other readers of your book, I've become, with admiration and thankfulness, an enthusiastic fan of this blessed healing method!
With the first swallow of this wonderful beverage I felt a soothing abatement of my arthritis-conditioned stomatitis." *(144)*

"Since taking the fungus tea beverage, inflammation in the genital area, which has plagued me constantly for several years, no longer appears." *(154)*

"After an influenza attack two years ago I suffered from a constant unexplainable mucous discharge in my throat. After 8 days of drinking Kombucha it has already diminished considerably." *(182)*

"After acquaintances of mine convinced me of the effects of the beverage I've become plainly addicted to it. I arise every day around five o'clock, and can hardly wait until it's late enough for me to drink a glass of Kombucha. For at least ten years I've had such pain in my left upper chest, and until now no doctor has been able to pinpoint its origin. I'd begun to think of myself as an imaginary invalid. At every blood test I show a high blood sedimentation rate.
Since I've been drinking Kombucha the pain has almost completely disappeared. Only when I suspend taking it because I've temporarily run out does the pain gradually start to return." *(184)*

Colds

"Every morning I drank a glassful on an empty stomach; my metabolic dysfunction regressed. Both my purulent sniffles and my bronchitis eased off." *(51)*

"We drink the fungus tea with great enthusiasm. We're not suffering at present from any acute or chronic illnesses, and drink it more or less as a preventive. It agrees very well with us, and we've made the discovery that cold infections last but a brief while and then disappear. Ater a short time digestive problems also vanish." *(65)*

"I've owned the tea fungus for about æ of a year. I've remained completely free of colds since I've been drinking the tea regularly, in contrast to the time before then." *(77)*

Joints, Vertebrae

"Since September 1990 I've been enthusiastically drinking Kombucha beverage which I myself prepare, a glassful every morning. I learned about and obtained the fungus from an acquaintance whose mother had successfully combatted her joint discomfort with it." *(23)*

"I learned about Kombucha tea through my niece in Augsburg; after four months she's all well again. Her period of suffering, an especially painful deformation of her vertebrae, stole away all her joy of living; she could no longer practice her nursing profession. By pure chance she met in the supermarket an acquaintance who had similar trouble, and learned about Kombucha tea from her. Now she is so happy to be free of pain once again." *(89)*

"I've obtained the tea fungus. Its effect is terrific. My inelastic joints have become supple again, they're no longer as stiff as before." *(108)*

"I've read your Kombucha book with great interest. I'd already been drinking Kombucha for a year, and my joint troubles were gone. But now they seem to have returned. My pharmacist said that I should discontinue (the tea) for four weeks, then it will again have an improved effect." *(116)*

Gout

"I've been drinking this Kombucha tea for half a year. Previously I suffered from gout in my fingers, but my metabolism has improved so much through Kombucha that this affliction has been almost completely redressed." *(9)*

"I started preparing the Kombucha tea fungus two years ago. In order to be entirely certain about it, I also bought your booklet.
I suffered from poor circulation in my middle finger for many years. The nail was deformed and the nailbed always inflamed and purulent. Then I went to the doctor because I had pain in my toes and couldn't roll my feet. After a blood test and examination the doctor determined that I had gout.

"Medication banished the pain indeed, but when the effects wore off the pain returned. For this reason I stopped taking the medication; besides, I wanted to know whether Kombucha tea really helped. I felt relief after several weeks. and after three months the doctor again made a blood analysis. He was quite astonished to find the various value-levels so good.

My finger is once again OK, and I no longer have gout troubles. The Kombucha fungus has helped me wonderfully!" *(142)*

"I suffered for eight years from gout in my feet. Last year I began a Kombucha cure. A marked dehydrating effect was the first result, and since then my gout troubles are scarcely worth mention-ing. When one thinks that I often had such really terrible pain before this cure, and that no other measures helped to end that pain." *(165)*

"Due to severe gout I could only venture forth with the help of a cane. After three months my state of health improved so drastically that I'm now completely pain-free." *(168)*

"I can joyfully inform you that Kombucha drops not only banish gout, but that my bowels work better since I've taken them." *(171)*

"My husband drinks Kombucha as if it were brook water, and since he does so has (without tablets) no more gout attacks." *(179)*

Glaucoma

"A few months ago I purchased a Kombucha fungus and prepared it according to Dr. Sklenar's directions. Yesterday in the health food store, when I inquired which sorts of tea were suitable for preparing the fungus, I was told that they no longer carry any articles which are associated with the Kombucha fungus, as its effect on human health is controversial. I myself have until now been unable to detect anything detrimental. Have shop personnel gone so far, perhaps, as to maintain that it's injurious to health? Surely you can explain to me why the beneficial effects of the fungus are now put in doubt.

I have glaucoma together with cataracts, and have discovered to my joy that the cataracts in my field of vision have diminished." *(42)*

Skin Problems

"After four weeks of drinking (Kombucha tea) regularly, my large-pored skin problem has normalized. A colleague of mine complained about her flame-red skin blemishes; these disappeared almost completely after two months.

We're all very happy about this super remedy, which tastes good into the bargain." *(88)*

"I've been drinking Kombucha tea for two months now, and can already observe that my acne condition (I'm 28 years old) is greatly improved, indeed that the skin has become smoother and finer-pored." *(114)*

"A short time ago I obtained a Kombucha fungus from an acquaintance. With it she had successfully healed a years-long skin allergy." *(152)*

Hope

"Please send me the recipe for preparing the fungus tea Kombucha. I have bacteria in my throat, pains in my body, nodules on my fingers, etc. The doctors say I'm not sick. I'd still like to drink the Kombucha beverage for reasons of health." *(115)*

Cancer

"I was operated on for an ovarian carcinoma in January 1992, and since summer of that year I've been drinking a liter of Kombucha fungus tea daily. My condition was excellent even during the chemotherapy, my blood also, so that I could undergo therapy. I'm convinced that it all can be attributed to the Kombucha fungus." *(7)*

"My husband and I have been drinking Kombucha tea since 1986, about a fifth of a liter daily. My husband had testicular cancer in 1984, underwent two serious operations followed by chemotherapy. Afterward we began to drink the tea, and up until now I have the impression that it's been beneficial, especially for my husband." (10)

"I've known since 1988 that I have intestinal cancer. This was also confirmed by blood tests performed pursuant to Dr. Sklenar, according to which I was in the second to third stage. It was becoming ever more troubling in September 1988. Indeed, I can eat everything, but I have a strong aversion to meat and sausage, and have suddenly lost eleven kilograms. I'm physically very weak, and cannot do any work. My blood is quite poor, especially in lack of iron. I have no appetite, but am constantly hungry.

I've been drinking a double shot glass of Kombucha tea three times daily for the past month; also Mutaflor. Now I also want to get Gelumoral rd. According to your book I should also be taking Kombucha drops. Indeed, I've already gained back two kilograms through the Kombucha tea and am maintaining this weight, although my weakness hasn't gotten better." *(14)*

"I am ill with cancer, and have just read your book about the Kombucha fungus. I have my seventh course of chemotherapy behind me and I am not at all convinced about this method, for every course is a little like dying. Now I've been drinking Kombucha tea for about three weeks, and notice clearly that's it's going better with me. I'm wholly convinced about Kombucha tea, and would cease chemotherapy entirely if another doctor would so advise. Now my present doctor tells me that there is no other possibility but this chemotherapy, and for that reason I fear to discontinue it." *(19)*

"My wife was diagnosed with breast cancer in February 1987. She should have been operated on immediately, but she refused. She embarked on a fasting cure for 42 days according to the method of Rudolf Preuss. During it she became very thin, but regained her previous weight after about three months. The nodes in her breast have until now gotten neither smaller nor larger. For two months she's been drinking two shot-glassfuls of Kombucha beverage three times daily. She'd already had years-long problems with delayed digestion With the Kombucha tea this condition has improved." *(26)*

"My mom got your book 'Tea Fungus Kombucha' from a fellow patient who lay in the same ward. Her husband had been diagnosed with testicular cancer twelve years ago; in addition to radiation, he's been drinking Kombucha tea for those same twelve years. He feels excellent healthwise and can no longer live without the tea." *(117)*

"I've been drinking Kombucha tea daily since my intestinal operation (cancer), and I believe that it has helped me very, very much. I feel well, and have no health problems of any kind." *(173)*

"I had to have an abdominal operation, for I was ill with cancer of the uterus. After subsequent radiation therapy I didn't feel well at all. I had a bad blood count and severe intestinal disorder. Since I've been drinking Kombucha tea I feel better every day; my blood count improves from week to week, and my elimination has normalized. I'm once again in good condition healthwise and have recovered very well. I take no other medication. According to my last hospital examination, I'm completely healthy." *(175)*

"I had cancer in the initial stage, and by taking Kombucha not only was I freed from suffering but now feel more capable and healthier than I did ten years ago." *(177)*

Leukemia

"I've had chronic leukemia since 1982. Since 1986 I've often had severe infections in my right cheek, and high fever. Doctors couldn't give me much help. I've had blood deficiency since January 1989; after each of several blood transfusions my blood supply would again decrease. I started taking the Kombucha fungus tea in May of 1989, and also take silicea once a day. Afterward I feel quite well, and my strength has also returned. The doctor is satisfied My infections have markedly diminished. (The doctor doesn't know that I drink Kombucha tea)." *(48)*

Stomach

"For some 22 years I've had persistent stomach ulcers. I've been drinking Kombucha fungus tea continuously for about three months. The beverage agrees with me very well; not only that, I've been since then almost entirely pain-free. My lay practitioner would forbid the fungus tea were it possible for him to do so." (40)

"I'd been suffering from gastritis for more than 20 years, and now I've been drinking Kombucha tea for the past five months with great success. I just spent three weeks abroad, and unfortunately didn't have the Kombucha with me; I feel my stomach trouble returning. I'm convinced, however, that I'll be OK again shortly or in a little longer time. Lucky for me that I got the fungus from friends." (47)

"Daily for the past six months I drink two wineglassfuls of the Kombucha fungus tea. And yet I have the utterly unusual feeling that I'm not able to get enough of it. I'm in my sixty-eighth year of life, and have already had stomach or intestinal troubles occasionally, also gastritis!
Since drinking Kombucha tea I no longer have the feeling that food simply plops into my stomach and then just lies there." (107)

"Three months ago I got a Kombucha fungus from an acquaint- ance, and since that time my husband and I drink the tea daily. I was at first rather unsure about it because of the acid, as I suffer from gastric trouble (heartburn), but to my amazement I have to state that the trouble has to a great extent decreased, even that it's outright disappeared." (133)

"In only a short time I was able to assert with certainty that this fungus heals gastritis." (164)

Migraine

"Two colleagues attained great success in combatting their migraine by treating it with the Kombucha beverage." (90)

"I suffered terribly from headaches. After about a half-year of drinking the tea I realize that I hardly have headaches any more.
I'm of the firm opinion that I'm better because of the Kombucha tea." (91)
"I'd like to say the following regarding your wonderful Kombucha tea: I'm sixty-five years old and have suffered for thirty-five years from

fearful headaches . . . After three months of Kombucha I no longer have any headaches. I'm overjoyed, for before no one could help me, only powders; now I no longer need powders." *(163)*

Morbus Crohn (Crohn's Disease)

"Can one treat Crohn's disease with Russian tea or must one necessarily take medicinal herbs against intestinal illnesses? For each liter I use 150 grams (5.3 oz.) of crystal sugar, but it makes the beverage taste too sweet. My neighbor, a woman whom I greatly honor and revere, is getting significantly better. Namely, she suffers from Crohn's disease, a dangerous almost incurable intestinal disorder where the bowels become covered with furuncles which in the end stages eat their way up to the throat. I suspect that Crohn's disease is a type of cancer, for cancer can have a hundred different names. Then (when it's called by another name) the patient maintains the illusion that hope is alive, and that he/she is not ill with cancer. I thank you from the bottom of my heart for the marvelous book you've written." *(135)*

Multiple Sclerosis

"Six months ago I discovered that my daughter is ill with MS. It was recommended to us that we treat this illness with the Kombucha fungus. We were able to obtain one from an acquaintance, and prepared the tea as follows: one tablespoon black tea to a liter of water, one scant handful of marigolds, one tablespoon hawthorn, and 100 grams (3.5 oz.) of sugar. This was very good from the beginning, and my daughter quickly felt the effects   Pain increased in her knees at first, but then it eased and they became supple." *(13)*

"I got your publication from a nephew who has been severely ill with MS for eleven years. He also believes that his illness has been alleviated by the fungus tea." *(153)*

Kidneys

"We treasure Kombucha highly; it helped my mother's kidney trouble and so far has spared her from dialysis." *(24)*

"I'm presently taking a Kombucha cure, for I have angina pectoris, too high blood pressure, and a likewise elevated cholesterol level. Up till now I've been able to determine that Kombucha has a strong diuretic effect, which may operate beneficially on my over- weight problem." *(145)*

Varicose Ulcer

"We've already been drinking Kombucha tea for almost four years; it agrees with us very well. You know, I'm not a hypochondriac nor a pill-swallower; I've always been in favor of natural cures, therefore the Kombucha suits us well. One of our daughters has a varicose ulcer. Well, she tried of her own accord, for want of any other advice, to apply a fungus over the wound. In this way she healed the leg. I've also tried treating other lesions with Kombucha and been successful." *(36)*

Rheumatoid Arthritis

"My wife and I have been taking the natural remedy Kombucha for some eighteen months, with measurable success.

At any rate, my wife, in spite of severe chronic rheumatoid arthritis and a dreadful period in a wheel chair, has come so far along with the aid of naturopathy that she can occasionally almost completely forget her malady. We want to thank you from our hearts for your commitment and for disseminating this knowledge." *(110)*

Rheumatism

"The rheumatic nodules which covered my fingers profusely have anyhow grown much smaller, although I've been taking no (other) medication for them. Kombucha must have helped there also." (172)

"Effects of the prepared tea are often amazing. For example, my seventy-three-year-old mother's rheumatoid arthritis abated within a few weeks." *(181)*

Thyroid

"I've been drinking Kombucha tea for about eight weeks now, naturally prepared by myself, and my thyroid discomfort (pressure on the throat) has markedly decreased. My nerves are also much better." *(155)*

Pain

"I encountered Kombucha recently through acquaintances and also in the bookstore by way of your book about the fungus tea. I've already noted that the beverage agrees with me very well. Incipient arthritis pain in my finger joint has gone, I can urinate better, and have less pain in my lymph channels, armpits and groin." *(42)*

"I've had pain in my hands and arms for many months now. I got a Kombucha fungus from a friend, and I've been drinking a small glassful of the tea daily for twenty days. In two days my pain had disappeared; I'm happy over that, and hope it stays that way." *(140)*

"I'm indeed so satisfied with Kombucha; since I've been drinking the tea everything is going much better with me. I'm no longer suffering so-
-the pain was becoming unbearable. My stomach is quite sensitive to powders, but your Kombucha has helped me immensely. My heartfelt thanks!" *(143)*

Vertigo, Nerves, Loss of Concentration

"About three months ago I received a gelatinous fungus as a gift. Well, after three months of drinking tea made from it I remark a considerable improvement in my afflictions (dizziness, nervousness, inability to concentrate)." *(4)*

"To a great extent I've lost my feelings of dizziness since I've been drinking Kombucha tea. Myself, I'm convinced that it's an item of outstanding excellence." *(5)*

"By and large, the tea has actually very much improved the general state of health of all of us. My wife lost her feelings of vertigo early on." *(96)*

"I've discerned that since my children have been drinking the fungus tea that they have more and longer perseverance in studying. And since I've been drinking your tea I can better endure my mother-in-law's daily onslaughts." *(150)*

"A year ago my son had a serious traffic accident with severe head injuries. As he was unconscious for a long period of time and subsequently had great difficulty in concentrating, I gave him your Kombucha drops for better oxygen intake. His condition has improved so much that he can take up his studies again, which back then he wouldn't have ventured to do." *(176)*

Digestion, Metabolism

"I'm a real fan of Kombucha tea and drink a small glassful regularly three times a day. My family also drinks Kombucha. The beverage refreshes me -- I feel energetic and can move my bowels marvelously. I'm also convinced of the positive effect of Kombucha tea on my metabolism." *(16)*

"Up till now I have imbibed two bottles of ready-to-drink Kombucha tea, and have had normal digestion for the first time in years (otherwise mostly liquid or pulpy). However, I can't afford a bottle per week at the store price, so I have infused the tea myself. But my attempts don't have the same results, although I was successful in cultivating the fungus from the flakes remaining in the two bottles." *(25)*

"I read your book about the Kombucha tea fungus with great interest. I also possess the tea fungus. For the past fourteen days I have regularly taken 1/8 liter of Kombucha tea morning and evening; the result was a marvelous bowel movement. But I must add that for the past six or seven years I have been a strict vegetarian." *(27)*

"I've been drinking the Kombucha beverage for about æ of a year. I had trouble with my gall bladder and with my digestion, troubles which have meanwhile gotten better." *(31)*

"I've owned a Kombucha tea fungus for three weeks, and in this short time have become habituated to the excellent beverage. My digestive troubles have already gotten better." *(35)*

"I am ill with cancer. I began the Kombucha cure one week ago, and feel very well since then, chiefly in the abdominal region." *(41)*

"I've been drinking Kombucha tea for four months because of my faulty immune system. Besides that, I've always had irksome intestinal trouble -- gas and stomach cramps, and very often diarrhea. The latter trouble has regressed and I no longer have a gas-distended stomach, though I do suffer back pain quite often." *(58)*

"My daughter has been drinking Kombucha tea for a year and it agre-es with her very well. Now, because of digestive trouble and over-weight, I have started with it. My digestion improved right away, but I'm concerned about my overweight, as the tea contains a large amount of sugar." *(59)*

"I've drunk Kombucha fungus tea for about three months, and the digestive troubles I've had for years seem to have been almost entirely eliminated." *(60)*

"We've been drinking the Kombucha beverage for some time and have already discovered its beneficial effects; namely, increased feel-ings of well-being and also improved condition of our stools (intestinal flora)." *(62)*

"My problems are digestive difficulties and severe, painful gas pockets (colonic irritation). I began this beverage cure for three days, but unfortunately had to break it off, for I got violent gas pains, worse than I'd had before. Can you advise me as to the cause of this reaction?" *(68)*

"I'd like to inform you that since I've been giving her the Mutaflor tablets, my 7 1/2-year-old daughter has rosy cheeks again, although increased flatulence too. Now I've also been giving her Kombucha drops; she's gotten much better and interests herself in everything much more." (69)

"I obtained a Kombucha tea fungus from a friend and started drinking the tea (it tastes very good). I felt well on the first day, but after that my stomach began to revolt, with watery stools and flatulence. I suffer from digestive upsets, tend to be constipated, have slow, burdensome digestion. I can't tolerate cabbage, eggs, sour milk, legumes, onions or anything cooked or fried in fat. I no longer eat meat. I've had to give up sourdough (rye) bread--only wheat bread is digestible. Now I've helped myself by diluting the Kombucha brew with spring water; it was too strong taken straight.
I already feel much better, can even drink milk again. I take Mutaflor as well." (70)

"Over the past three years I've drunk a total of 4 to 5 thousand liters of Kombucha tea, a liqueur glassful at a time, and my constant headaches have become appreciably milder. I also had terrible gas and constipation, and tried everything including flaxseed and wheat bran without success. Now I drink one or two shot glasses of Kombucha on an empty stomach, and my gas and constipation problems are nearly gone. Also, the painful abdominal twinges (which ostensibly derive from a cyst) have become in the past three days less intense. This 'ostensibly' relates to assertions from four different doctors; two of them maintain that there is a cyst; one says he simply feels that one ovary is slightly larger and there's a prolapsed bladder, and the fourth doctor says that I'm in perfect health, that I'm only imagining the pain." (76)

"The beverage tastes excellent to me, and I also notice its effect, especially regarding my digestion!" (78)

"We have read your book 'Tea Fungus Kombucha' with great diligence. In the past five weeks my husband has undergone three operations--prostate carcinoma, kidneys, and then suddenly a purulent gall bladder had to be removed. At the same time liver metastasis was discovered. The medical verdict: Not a chance! For ten days now he's been taking the preparations recommended by Dr. Sklenar, together with daily injections of Colibiogen ampoules. His bowel functions are once again in order." (79)

"For three months I've been drinking Kombucha fungus tea, which I enthusiastically recommend to others. After two weeks I enjoyed regular elimination, up to twice a day. Previously I could move my bowels only once a week." (88)

"We got hold of a copy of the Kombucha (book) and now, after drinking (the tea) regularly have attained improvement in mouth-, stomach- and intestinal flora." (97)

"I got a Kombucha fungus from a night-watch attendant, and drink the tea daily, which agrees with me very well. I take Mutaflor for my multiple sclerosis. I had lots of gas with the first capsules, but now it's going much better with me. I must say in addition that I've also been taking laxatives for almost thirty years. In spite of the fungus tea and Mutaflor, I still require a laxative, but less of it. Twice I even went without it." (101)

"I've read your book with great interest. My four-year-old son has been drinking Kombucha tea for two months (constipation of psychological origin), and has improved somewhat without other medication (Bibiteral). He gets a glassful each day. Can I give him more of it than that?" (81)

"I obtained the Kombucha tea through an acquaintance. I suffer from chronic constipation and have always taken teas and tablets. My digestion has improved every day through Kombucha tea." (84)

"About twelve weeks ago I was diagnosed with the rare metabolic disorder Porphyria Cutana-tarda. The malady is treated with venesection therapy. I've been drinking Kombucha tea I prepare myself for about twenty weeks. I very much like to drink this beverage and want to continue drinking it, for I 've alread noticed some slight success." (100)

"I've suffered from intestinal dysfunction for years. Now, thank God, only to a lesser degree, for I've obtained some good drops from a lay practitioner. Kombucha tea agrees very well with me. My husband also drinks it, diluted, not for health reasons as I do, but rather because it tastes good to him." *(104)*

"I had bowel-movement problems for long years -- without laxative pills I couldn't go at all. In three months I've eliminated this affliction by the drink cure. On the whole, one feels better ." *(109)*

"I'm an enthusiastic drinker of Kombucha tea and have the feeling that it works very well against gas and stomach upsets." *(124)*

"For a good year my husband and I have drunk Kombucha tea according to Dr. Sklenar. Since then we've noticed improvement in our digestive processes." *(122)*

"I'm 66 years old, healthy up till now, and I live healthwise in accord with general knowledge. Since I've been drinking Kombucha tea I've had regular bowel movements, which I never had before. That's tangible proof that the tea works." *(103)*

"I've already been utilizing the Kombucha tea for a long time without thinking of it even remotely as a cancer preventive. I got it from acquaintances who thought I should try it out against my many gas problems, which could be attributed to improper diet (too sweet and too greasy) during my student days. Truth to tell, my 'wind' diminishes when I go through with a Kombucha cure, so I keep taking it over and over again." *(125)*

"For many years I've had persistent gas pains. They exert pressure on my back up to the shoulder blades and stabbing pains against my heart. I must always take tablets or Hetterich drops. I've been to many lay practitioners, but no one can tell me the origin of these weird gas troubles. I got some relief from kefir made from milk, which I prepared myself. I've been drinking Kombucha tea for six months now, and it's eased my stomach pains, bowel movements and gas attacks." *(127)*

"After an infection with Yersin's bacteria I had intestinal troubles for many years and am still undergoing medical treatment. The principal symptoms are: constipation, enzyme deficiency, severe gas pains in the epigastric region, and fatigue. I've been drinking Kombucha tea for 1/2-year and since then feel generally better." *(131)*

74

"A few months ago I obtained through happy chance a precious Kombucha fungus. I treasure it greatly and take care of it, for we've had positive success with it indeed: our children are glad about their improved digestion, my husband has regular bowel movements, and I have fewer gas problems." *(136)*

"I read your booklet, got interested in Kombucha fungus, and prepared the tea myself. With it I noted a marked improvement in my general condition; the intestinal flora which were always troubling before (in spite of Symbioflor treatment) have normalized." *(148)*

"I've drunk the tea for three weeks now, and could immediately observe an improvement in my digestion. I'm over eighty years old, live without a gall bladder, and now have, apart from intervertebral disk pain, high blood pressure and rheumatism. About eight days after starting to take the tea my pulse started racing, and I ask myself whether the black tea I use in preparing the fungus is proper for me. Otherwise I've always drunk herb tea, which is suitable for my state of health. My doctor is a classical physician, and is no friend of the tea fungus. I've gotten pills for the high blood pressure and digitalis for the rapid pulse. After other patients found that when they took Kombucha tea other medications were no longer necessary, I would also be happy to enter this happy state!" *(149)*

"Since the time I had to undergo an abdominal operation ten years ago (I was then 29 years old), I had problems with elimination. Since I've been drinking your fungus tea, my bowel movements are normal again." *(151)*

"I had intestinal troubles for many years, couldn't move my bowels without taking laxatives. I started drinking Kombucha tea, and after a half year found that laxatives were no longer needed. My blood count has also improved." *(174)*

Vitality, Well-being

"I've been drinking Kombucha for about two months and feel very energetic and receptive. My acquaintances are also enthusiastic about this beverage." (3)

"I received a Kombucha fungus as a gift about two years ago, recommended as a personal tip. I immediately and enthusiastically included it in my diet. Not only does it have an excellent taste, it also seems to have beneficial effects on me in many ways." (21)

"Please send me your book about the Kombucha fungus tea. The only thing I really know is that it has a superlative effect on me and that I simply need it." (37)

"I'm seventy-two years old and still engage in running sports (running in place). It's important that one should already start drinking Kombucha tea months before he takes up this running activity. The fungus tea strengthens the leg muscles. That's not a doctor's opinion but my own; that's what I myself have done, and gotten along well by it (running) up till now." (38)

"My family and I have already sensed a quite positive effect in a very short time." (92)

"My wife and I have been drinking Kombucha tea regularly, tea we ourselves prepare, for several months. We've already concluded that it has beneficial effects on our general state of health." (99)

"We've been drinking Kombucha tea regularly for the past three years. It agrees with us exceptionally well." (112)

"I've been drinking Kombucha daily for two months and feel well all-around. I was even able to convince my husband." (120)

"We've been drinking Kombucha tea for about two years. and it has regularized our state of health very well." (141)

"My fungus has grown larger. I drink Kombucha with enthusiasm and feel myself to be decidedly more energetic than before." (146)

"A while back our daughter obtained a Kombucha fungus from one of her woman friends. She drank the beverage regularly over a several-week period and it made her feel very well. This fact induced her to commend the fungus to us, her parents." (17)

Side Effects

". . . came into possession of a Kombucha fungus. I observe a marked freshening of body and spirit. I'm rather unsure about its preparation. I use cane sugar for sweetening, but sometimes find the drink too sweet. A side phenomenon is periodic flatulence!" (1)

"I suffer from chronic lymphatic leukemia which was diagnosed four years ago. For about six weeks I've also been treating the illness with Kombucha, Mutaflor and Gelum oral-rd. This additional treat- ment agrees well with me. Only I have the impression that the lymph glands in my neck and in my groin have become somewhat harder. My family doctor is also of this opinion." (2)

"I've possessed this tea fungus for some time, and after enjoying it had to observe on the same evening an unpleasant manifestation. I had quite severe flatulence and abdominal pains the whole night through, and diarrhea on the day following." (11)

"I've been drinking Kombucha regularly for some time and it agrees with me very well, but I have the feeling that it's causing a slight increase in weight."(12)

"I'm writing to you because I have a great problem. I drank self- prepared Kombucha tea for about ten days. Suddenly I broke out in a rash. I didn't drink Kombucha tea for five days; the rash disappeared completely after three days. After six more days had passed I started to drink Kombucha again, and on the third day of drinking it the rash began again." (28)

"As I have been drinking Kombucha tea for a long time and have had good results with it, I recommended it to an elderly woman who has also been drinking it for a long time now. The woman abruptly informed me that she got diarrhea and a rash outbreak accompanied by itching. This woman had gall bladder and stomach operations about fifteen or twenty years ago." (29)

"I got a Kombucha fungus about three months ago. At first I prepared the tea with 100 grams sugar to one liter of tea (a mixture of fruit, rose hips, peppermint and black teas), and changed it after seven days. But the beverage caused unbearable phenomena in the form of severe flatulence and stomach pains. Thereafter I prepared the tea with honey instead of sugar (100 g honey to 1 l tea) and behold, my innards tolerate the tea wonderfully. The fungus also seems to like honey, for it constantly increases in size." *(50)*

"I've drunk Kombucha for some time, and I'm wholly enthusiastic about it. Unfortunately, my weight is increasing. Can one prepare Kombucha with less sugar, or even none at all?" *(52)*

"I've been drinking Kombucha tea for eight days now and today was shocked to discover that I've gained two kilograms (4 1/2 lb.). I've suffered with thyroid trouble for twenty years and take thyroxin daily. My doctor says I take too high a dose, but I'm loath to decrease it, for then my weight steadily increases. Attempts to reduce haven't succeeded in years." *(53)*

"With me it's a matter of chronic herpes zoster (shingles) without skin eruptions, probably brought about through polyneuritis, for I suffer from severe neuralgic pains over my entire body, and have the feeling that they're getting progressively worse. My vital organs are also chronically inflamed. I drink 3/4 of a liter Kombucha tea daily, but have now discontinued it, as I discovered, unfortunately, that it made my gastritis worse. I was naturally quite sorry about that, for in one regard I'd experienced its detoxifying effects. My head has become much clearer and I have dreams once again. And I'm no longer as fatigued as before. I regularly drink diluted Kombucha drops, which agree well with me." *(80)*

"I've been taking three glasses of Kombucha tea daily for three months, to foster cartilage-development and for weakness in connective tissue brought on by rheumatism remedies. Several times shingles resulted. For about the past three weeks I've had an itchy, burning skin and the inception of pimples and blisters, chiefly on the elbows and in the armpits as well as on the chest area. Question: Can this be attributed to the drinking of Kombucha tea? Or are the toxins eliminated by it?" *(87)*

"Since I've been drinking Kombucha tea, daily for about the past five weeks (about four liters over ten days), I've discovered that it leads to weight increase. As I tend to gain anyway, I must always pay heed to my weight (I'm 55 years old, have Hepatitis B and only one kidney). Can one prepare Kombucha with something else instead of sugar?" *(123)*

"We've been preparing Kombucha tea for half a year; it tastes very good to us. But we've gained several kilograms in body weight. Can this be attributed to the Kombucha tea?" *(30)*

"I must dilute the Kombucha tea, but solely with 'Fachinger', otherwise I have stomach problems." *(106)*

"After a brief period I can already impart a success story. My body weight has 'automatically' sharply decreased, without the strain of the otherwise customary diet." *(129)*

"My husband and I are each fifty-six years old. We've been drinking self-prepared Kombucha tea enthusiastically for some three months. Is it possible that our weight gain is due to the beverage? We're constantly battling overweight (my husband about nine kilograms, myself five kilos). My husband drinks (Kombucha) because of rheumatism. Since my twelfth year I can't go to the toilet without Agiolax." *(130)*

"Since I've been drinking Kombucha tea I've gotten numerous pimples and other skin blemishes on my face. As I've ingested scarcely any sugar, coffee or alcohol for a long time, I've become somewhat mistrustful about the beverage, for it tastes so good that I've drunk quite a lot of it!" *(132)*

Conclusion

Research by *Enderlein* provided the answer more than 60 years ago that only biological means – Kombucha is one – can be successful remedies in cases of cancer. The cancer virus "Endobiont", "Siphonospora polymorpha" or whatever name it may be given, can only be defeated by depriving it of its nutrient substratum – its environment. *Pasteur* already knew:

"The microbe is nothing, the terrain (environment) is everything!"

And eminent natural practitioners, such as *Louis Kühne,* said: "An acute disease is unthinkable unless it was preceded by a strain on the body through foreign substances." Therefore the most fundamental principle of any natural treatment must be the elimination of toxic wastes from the organism, so that a healthy environment with strong powers of resistance can be restored!

The Kombucha fungus sprouts in an acidic environment and thus eliminates, or retards in its development, the primitive microbe "Endobiont", which thrives in an alkaline environment, and thus renders or keeps it harmless for man. The treatment of cancer as well as of precancerous stages including tumors, has a simple key:

Fungus vs. fungus!

Of course, extensive research will still have to be conducted, but the therapy according to Sklenar in cases of metabolic diseases and cancer with the proven natural remedy "Kombucha" as well as colicines is pointing a helpful way. So far, success has proven him right! Maybe some day microbiologists and pharmacologists will be able to isolate the active agents of Kombucha with its bacterial metabolic products, so that a serum can be developed which through inoculation will deliver mankind from this dreadful scourge.

As long as the knowledge concerning the existence of a cancer virus is shared by only a few doctors, so that the theory concerning the causative organism does not manifest itself in cancer therapy, cancer will not be conquered.

In light of this, the smallest knot in the breast already constitutes a growth and is no longer a precancerous phenomenon. This is by no means an early diagnosis. Only when the 'misfortune' measures an inch or so, will it be correctly diagnosed and treated by chemotherapy and rays or operated on. At this stage, however, cancer therapy is unsatisfactory for several reasons, as past experience has shown:

- During surgery primary foci and proud flesh are removed, but metastases remain unharmed. Moreover, in the course of operations large amounts of noxious substances are released from tumor tissues, with which the body cannot cope, so that death may ensue.

- Also ray therapy has not been able to fulfill its expectations. Same as surgery, it leaves injuries such as burns in healthy tissue. This makes for another weak point in the organism. Moreover it should be noted that a virus with a resistance far superior to man's cannot be conquered by even the most refined means of modern technology.

- Last, but not least, not one chemotherapeutical remedy has so far proved effective against cancer. On the contrary, the accumulation of chemical waste products in the body weakens its resistance even more. After the euphoria surrounding the "miracle cancer drug interferon" has subsided, the pointed question remains unanswered why interferon was extolled as a "remedy against viruses". On which considerations and research findings is such a theory based which says that a "remedy aigainst viruses" can constitue the breakthrough in the battle against cancer?

Finally a remark to the question why one organ may more easily be affected by cancer than another: The illness will always break out at the weakest part of the organism. Just like a chain is only as strong as its weakest link, the human body is only as healthy as its weakest organ.

In conclusion, here is an annotation concerning the future of AIDS. As *Dr. Sklenar* stated in his introductory essay, the viruses discovered by Gallo, Montagnier, v. Brehmer, Scheller, Enderlein, Sklenar et al. are identical. AIDS as a disease between whose infection and outbreak years can pass has been decoded. The initial symptoms of the ailment are feebleness, fever, diarrhea, weight loss and, later on, severe organic disturbances. All AIDS patients suffer from the same peculiar immune defect. Obviously, the symptoms of AIDS are also to a large extent identical with cancer symptoms.

Dr. Luc Montagnier from the Pasteur Institute in Paris found the "Lymphademopathic Virus" (LAV), and nobody doubts any longer that this is the AIDS virus. A little later, *Dr. Robert C. Gallo* from the American Cancer Institute in Bethesda, Maryland, isolated the "Human-T-Lymphodropic Virus" (HTLV), and nobody doubts any longer that these two viruses are identical. Here AIDS, there cancer – with one and the same virus!

If according to present knowledge AIDS patients should not donate blood, then why should cancer patients? In every single case donated blood ought to be examined to determine the development stage of potential blood parasites and soon the pH-value of the blood should be measured at every examination.

P.S.: For further information, criticism and suggestions please write (with return postage) to:

Ms. Rosina Fasching
Post Box 98
A-9021 Klagenfurt
Austria

Appendix

Aetiopathogenesis	– cause of a disease
alkalinity	– alkaline content of a solution
amoeboid	– changeable, transforming
antibiotics	– collective term for agents which impede or arrest the growth and development of bacteria. The most important antibiotics are obtained from fungus cultures (penicillin, streptomycin, neomycin)
arteriosclerosis	– degenerative changes of arteries, arteriosteogenesis
bilirubin	– red dye of the gall
biological	– concerning living organisms
chemotherapy	– treatment of infectious diseases with chemical substances which impede the growth of, or kill viruses, e.g. antibiotics and sulfonamides
chronic	– proceeding slowly (as opposed to: acute)
dehydration	– withdrawal of water
divergent	– deviating, separating (opposite: convergent)
electrolytic balance	– assimilation, effect and excretion of electrolytes, the most important being sodium, potassium, calcium and magnesium
elimination	– removal; here: devitalizing
erythrocytes	– red blood corpuscles

furunculosis	– painful festering inflammation of the sebaceous glands all over the body
gastritis	– stomach ailment, inflammation of the stomach, especially its mucous membranes
genesis	– origin, development (of a disease)
homeopathy	– method of treatment employing remedies in a highly diluted form, which in a healthy person would produce the very symptoms that the patient already has. Opposite: allopathy
immunize	– make resistant through inoculation
immune system	– the body's defensive system against germs, with the formation of antibodies being crucial
in vitro (Latin 'in the glass')	– in a test tube, performed in the laboratory (experiment)
carcinogenic	– cancer-producing, cancer-causing
latent	– concealed; existing but not apparent
malignant	– likely to cause death
megalocytes	– degenerated, bloated red blood corpuscles
metabolism	– assimilation of nutrients and oxygen, excretion of non-organic and noxious substances
metastasis	– spread, displacement. Appearance of secondary growths in other parts of the body
micro-organism	– tiniest living things, microbes
mitochondria	– protoplasma parts essential for the cell's energy balance
morphological	– concerning form and shape
parabiosis	– cohabitation of two individuals grown together, e. g. Siamese twins
parasite	– organism living at the expense of others, e. g. bacteria, viruses, fungi and worms
pharmacology	– science of drugs

pathological	– degenerate, causing illness
physiological	– concerning normal living functions
pH-level	– concentration level of hydrogen ions
precancerosis	– stage preceding cancer; disease which may lead to cancer, e. g. a stomach ulcer preceding stomach cancer
prevention	– prophylaxis, guarding against
prophylactic	– preventive measures to ward off a disease
prothrombin synthesis	– accumulation of enzymes enhancing the coagulation of blood
protozoon	– single-cell organism
resorption	– assimilation of liquid or solid matter in comminuted form into tissue liquids, mainly blood
sanitation	– here: restitution of health
symbiosis	– cohabitation of different organisms for mutual benefit
therapeuticum	– remedy
urobilin	– gall dye in the urine. Increased urobilin content in the urine is an important indication of disease, e. g. concerning liver and gall
virus	– minute causative agent

COLORED PICTURE
SECTION

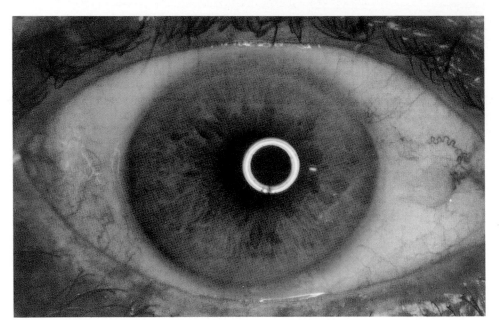

Specimen 1: *(right iris) – Round the iris ruffle (intestinal area) there is a fissured relief, which is a clue indicating metabolic diseases. Where digit 6 on a clock would be there is a rhombic defect with a tiny brown speck of pigment. This indicates that inflamed processes are under way in the areas of foot, knee, leg and kidney.*

Specimen 2: *(left iris) – Here again serious metabolic disturbances become evident (deposits of cholesterol and uric acid). The cholesterol pigments along the intestinal walls are quite striking. A large dark lacuna (transmutation of substance) in the right half near 'digit 3' indicates a former inflammation of the lungs. If striking or microscopic pigments are visible beside the substance defect, the disease is recent or only a few months old. Near '10' (nose) and '11' (frontal cavity) two striking brown pigment specks are visible.*

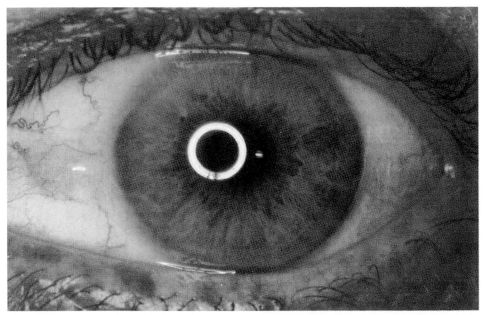

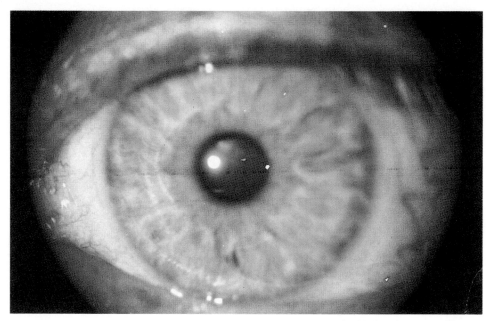

Specimen 3: *(left iris) – The grey and white stripes and knots indicate a considerable disturbance caused by uric acid. The brownish discolorations indicate cholesterol deposits. This is the typical manifestation of rheumatic ailments and gout. Loss of substance and the so-called cramp rings (intestinal cramps) indicate serious metabolic diseases.*

Specimen 4: *(right iris) – Here the broad, fissured intestinal relief strikes the viewer. The many arrow-like lines and the dark brown pigment speck indicate high cholesterol. The arrows pointing upwards are surrounded by minute, microscopic pigment dots, which indicates brain ailments. The iris has characteristic, large cramp rings which surround the intestinal area. The brown pigment spots indicate organic disturbances according to their topography (esophagus, thyroid gland, bowels, liver).*

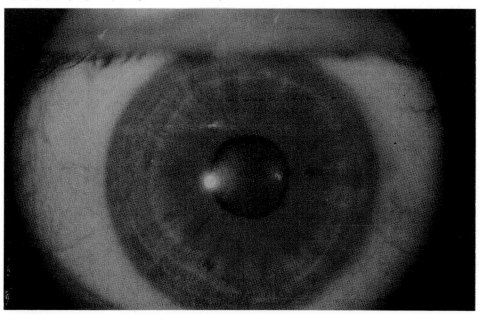

RIGHT IRIS

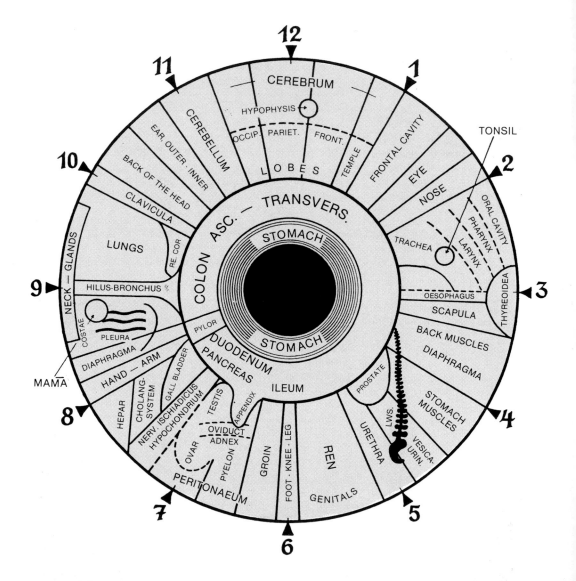

LEFT IRIS

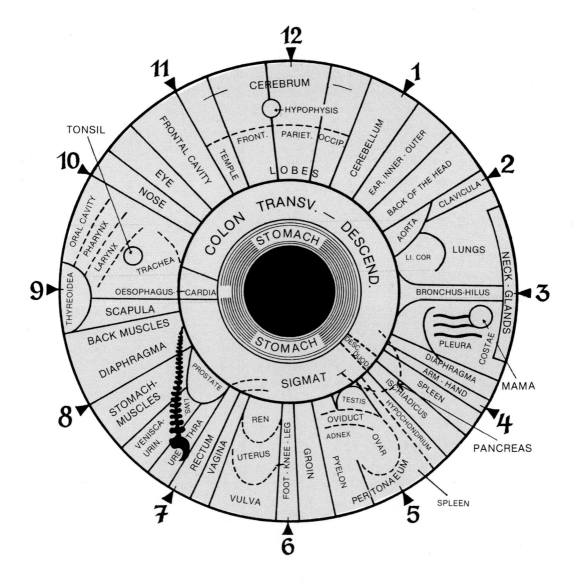

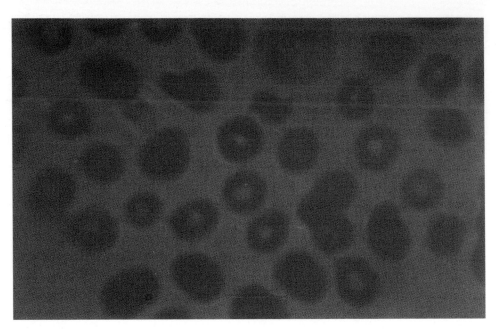

*The existence of degenerated, excrescent erythrocytes **(megalocytes)** indicates malignity.*

Stage 1:
*The blood parasite attacks the red blood corpuscles (erythrocytes). At first, only a few isolated spores and a slight damage of the erythrocytes are visible **(granula).***

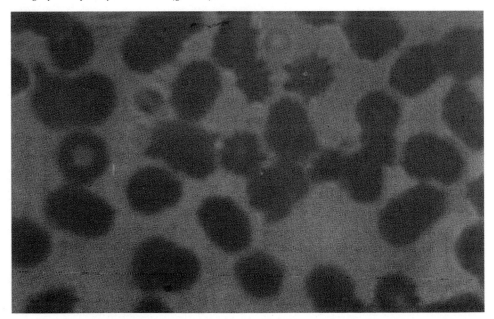

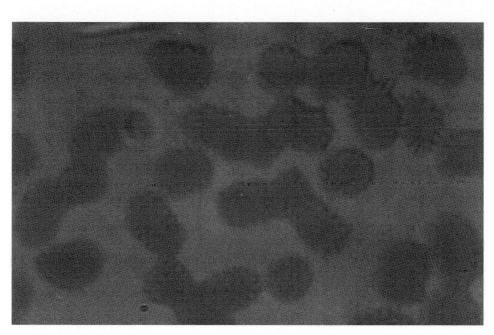

Stage 2:
*In precancerous cases, granula and **thorn-apple forms** are visible years before the appearance of a tumor.*

Stage 3:
*In the course of the disease, **blisters begin to form**.*

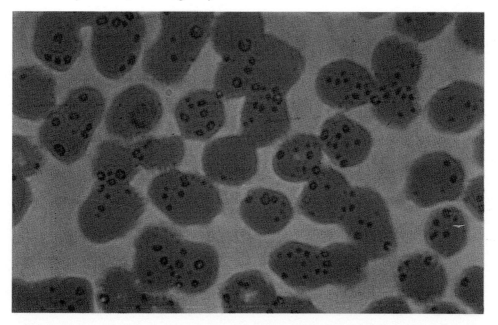

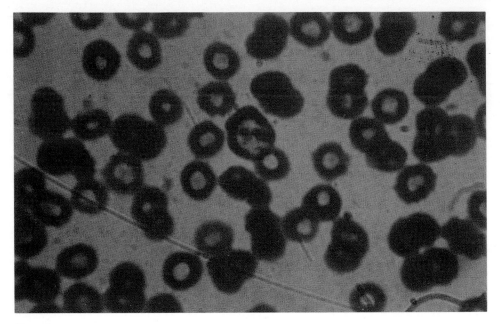

Stage 4:
*In advanced cases of tumors, the erythrocytes appear hollowed out and show marked loss of substance (**holes, ring shapes**).*